SKELETAL MATURITY
The Knee Joint as a Biological Indicator

NOTICE

A reproduction of Fig. 14 on transparent plastic to be used as outlined on pages 70-71 will be found in the back of the book. Replacement copies can be obtained from Dr. Alex Roche, The Fels Research Institute, Yellow Springs, Ohio 45387

SKELETAL MATURITY
The Knee Joint as a Biological Indicator

Alex F. Roche
The Fels Research Institute

and

Howard Wainer and David Thissen
The University of Chicago

PLENUM MEDICAL BOOK COMPANY • New York and London

Library of Congress Cataloging in Publication Data

Roche, Alex F   1921-
    Skeletal maturity.

    Bibliography: p.
    Includes index.
    1. Man—Age determination. 2. Knee-Aging. I. Wainer, Howard, joint author. II.
Thissen, David, joint author. III. Title. [DNLM: 1. Age determination by skeleton—
Methods—Collected works. 2. Knee joint—Growth and development—Collected
works. WE870 S627]
QP86.R55   573'.6'718   75-35927
ISBN 0-306-30900-9

"To record shape has been far
easier than to understand it."

C. S. Sherrington
Man and His Nature, Ed. 2
Cambridge University Press
1963, p. 99

Preface

Marked interest in the assessment of skeletal
maturity began for one of us (A.F.R.) when the late
Normand L. Hoerr provided a guest in his home with the
recently published Greulich-Pyle atlas, for light
reading. During the remainder of that year, S. Idell
Pyle fostered this interest by her continuous encourage-
ment and advice. The seed of interest, so effectively
planted and nurtured, has continued to grow for more
than 20 years.

Soon it was recognized that the existing atlases
should be modified; more gradually it was realized
that a completely new method of assessment of skeletal
maturity was needed. However, because of the sheer
size of the task, and the complexity of the concepts,
it was difficult to develop a new method. The possibility was considered over the years, but an attempt
was delayed because three elements were essential for
the successful implementation of a research plan.
The work could not be done without a large collection
of high quality serial radiographs; this was available
at The Fels Research Institute. Specialized statistical skills were needed to analyze sequential changes
in qualitative and quantitative indicators. These
skills were provided by the co-authors. The third necessary element (financial assistance) was made available by The National Institutes of Health, Bethesda,
Maryland through Grant HD-04629.

We wish to acknowledge the assistance of many
colleagues, particularly R. Darrell Bock and James R.

v

Murray of The University of Chicago and G. Frank
Johnson of The Dayton Children's Medical Center.
We are fortunate that the research assistants associated
with the study were so interested and intelligent.
Major contributions were made by Elma Barnes, Frances
Bodnar and Emily Townsend. In this field, illustrations
play an important part--the present ones were done by
Nancy Harvey. Dorothy Gross and Joan Hunter typed the
manuscript, not once but many times. Roy Acheson read
the manuscript critically and improved it in many ways.

We are grateful also for the help and support
given by the Member-Directors and Officers of the
Samuel S. Fels Fund of Philadelphia.

Despite all the help from those mentioned above,
this work would have been impossible without the
cooperation of those enrolled in The Fels Longitudinal
Study and the earlier contributions of many investigators, especially those who worked at The Brush Foundation in Cleveland, Ohio.

Alex F. Roche
Howard Wainer
David Thissen

Contents

GLOSSARY

<u>Apposition</u> -- a growth process involving addition to
   a surface.
<u>Chondrification</u> -- the process of cartilage formation.
<u>Chrondrocyte</u> -- a cartilage cell.
<u>Diaphysis</u> -- the shaft, or central portion, of a long
   or short bone.
<u>Discriminability</u> -- the slope of the fitted logistic
   junction, denoted b$_j$. This indicates the rapidity
   with which a particular indicator matures.
<u>Disseminated calcification</u> -- a condition in which
   diffuse radiographic shadows are present near
   the ossified part of the epiphysis with which
   they may be continuous.
<u>Dysharmonic maturation</u> -- the occurrence of markedly
   disparate maturity levels among the bones of an
   area within an individual.
<u>Endochondral</u> -- within cartilage. In the present
   context, this refers to the site of ossification.
<u>Epiphyseal zone</u> -- the cartilage between the epiphyseal
   center of ossification and the metaphysis.
<u>Epiphysis</u> -- the end of a long or short bone. Early
   it is cartilaginous, later ossification occurs in
   this cartilage.
<u>Maturity indicator</u> -- in the present context, a radio-
   graphically visible feature that assists the
   assessment of skeletal maturity.
<u>Metaphysis</u> -- the end of the diaphysis.
<u>Osteocyte</u> -- a bone cell.
<u>Perichondrium</u> -- a fibrous connective tissue that
   covers cartilage, except over articular surfaces.

<u>Periosteum</u> -- a fibrous layer that covers the surfaces
    of bones, except where tendons or ligaments are
    attached or where the surface of the bone is
    covered by cartilage.
<u>Skeletal age</u> -- a value assigned to a bone or skeletal
    area that is the level of maturity expressed in
    years and months.
<u>Subperiosteal</u> -- beneath the periosteum. In the present
    context, this refers to a site of ossification.
<u>Terminal plate</u> -- a layer of cortical bone, on the
    metaphyseal aspect of the epiphyseal center of
    ossification, that is visible radiographically.
<u>Threshold</u> -- for each grade of a maturity indicator,
    this is the age at which 50 percent of the indi-
    viduals are assigned that grade or a higher one.
<u>Trabeculae</u> -- thin pieces of cancellous bone.

CHAPTER I

INTRODUCTION

Children differ in their rates of maturation within the same sex and ethnic group. Consequently, children of the same chronological age may differ in measures of biological age. This is clear from the variations that occur, within age groups, in dental status and the development of secondary sex characters. Differences occur also in the rates of maturation of the skeleton; many of these changes can be recognized in radiographs. Early, a "bone" is not radio-opaque when it consists entirely of fibrous tissue and cartilage. As it matures, the radio-opaque ossified area extends into the cartilaginous model of the bone. These changes are visible radiographically and they are used to assess the maturity levels of bones or skeletal areas. Scales have been developed that allow, with some reservations as will be seen later, these subjective impressions of skeletal maturity level to be recorded in years of skeletal age. Less frequently, skeletal maturity scores are assigned to radiographs.

A bone-specific approach is necessary because, within individuals, there are differences among bones in the order of chondrification and ossification of diaphyses and centers of ossification in epiphyses and in the order of epiphyseo-diaphyseal fusion (Gardner and Gray, 1953; O'Rahilly and Meyer, 1956; Gardner et al., 1959; O'Rahilly et al., 1960; Garn et al., 1961; Roche, 1963; Roche et al., 1974).

It has been claimed that when there is a wide range of maturity between the bones of an area, its maturity level cannot be described adequately by a

1

single figure (Greulich and Pyle, 1959; Anderson, 1971).
Greulich and Pyle (1959) suggested recording the
maturity level appropriate for most of the bones and
the skeletal ages of those that were divergent.

This has been applied only rarely, in part because
of the lack of normative reference data. Recently,
however, the distributions of the ranges of bone-
specific skeletal ages (Greulich-Pyle) within individual
hand-wrists have been available for national probability
samples of United States children and youth (Roche
et al., 1974 and in press). The second limitation is
that the health-related significance of an unusually
wide range of bone-specific skeletal ages is unknown
except that it is found in a few uncommon diseases,
e.g., epiphyseal dysplasia and homocystinuria (Poznanski
et al., 1971). If such diseases are suspected, it is
certainly appropriate to record the extent to which
maturation is dysharmonic. The third limitation is that
the errors of the estimates of bone-specific skeletal
ages (and, for that matter, of area skeletal ages) are
unknown when the atlas method is applied. The atlas
method is described in more detail later (pp. 28-32).
Briefly, it consists in comparing the radiograph to be
assessed with a set of standards that represent approximate modal levels of maturity within chronological
age groups.

Using the method employed in the present study,
data from indicators at different maturity levels can
be combined statistically to a meaningful single figure
for an area. However, one aim of the present investigation was to obtain bone-specific skeletal ages for
the knee. The RWT method allows this but at most
maturity levels the errors of the estimates are too
large for these bone-specific skeletal ages to
be meaningful.

Usually, ratings of skeletal maturity are made of
the hand-wrist because its radiographic positioning is
simple and many bones are present in a small area. The
hand-wrist is no more and no less representative of the
whole skeleton than most other areas (Garn et al., 1964)

but it is less closely related to stature than the knee
(Todd, 1931).

Assessments of skeletal maturation are required
commonly in the clinical management of children with
deviant statures. Typically, these children have
unusual past or present rates of elongation at the knee
joint. Skeletal maturity levels of the knee are more
relevant than the corresponding levels for the hand-
wrist in the clinical management of such children. The
knee has one further advantage. The bones in this area
do not reach adult levels of maturity until comparatively late, whereas many of the hand-wrist bones,
particularly carpals and distal phalanges, become "adult"
at about 15 years in boys and 13 years in girls.

The new RWT (Roche, Wainer, Thissen) method of
assessing skeletal maturity differs from the best known
current methods (Greulich and Pyle, 1959; Tanner et al.,
1962, 1972, 1975) in the area assessed. It differs from
all previous methods in the nature of the observations
on which assessments are based, the provision of a range
of shapes to which some indicator grades can be assigned,
and in the statistical analyses used to construct the
new scale. The result is an increase in known validity,
an increase in the proportion of individuals for whom
assessments can be made (especially at younger ages)
and the provision, for the first time, of the errors of
the estimate for each individual.

The Need for Skeletal Age Assessments

In many genetically determined syndromes, the rates
and patterns of skeletal maturation differ from those
observed in healthy children. In children with such
syndromes, assessments of skeletal maturation assist
diagnosis and increase understanding of the skeletal
changes. In children with unusual statures, there is
often concern, on the part of child and parent, about
the deviant present stature and the possibility that
mature stature will be deviant. This concern can cause
adverse psychological effects, especially near the usual

age of puberty, when the statures of many short or tall children become increasingly deviant. Because of the close associations between skeletal elongation and skeletal maturation, the management of such children will be improved by skeletal age assessments that are more accurate than those possible previously and the accuracy of which is known.

These assessments are needed in order to select, from among children with deviant statures, those who should be treated, to regulate the dosage of the therapeutic agent and to estimate its effects on adult stature. Selection for therapy is particularly diffi-cult when the therapeutic agent is scarce, e.g., human growth hormone. Accurate predictions of adult stature, which are based in part on assessments of skeletal maturity (Bayley and Pinneau, 1952; Roche et al., 1975) are needed to identify those children most in need from a physical viewpoint. To take another example; an artificially induced pseudopuberty may be necessary in a girl with Turner's syndrome although this treatment may reduce her potential for growth in stature. The necessary clinical judgment should depend, in part, on estimates of skeletal maturity to determine her present status, her potential for further growth in stature and her estimated adult stature.

Some short children are treated with "anabolic" steroids that have high anabolic-androgenic ratios, when these are measured in experimental animals by the current unsatisfactory methods. These ratios are not accurate reflections of therapeutic effectiveness (Roche et al., 1963). When anabolic steroids are administered, their effects on the rate of skeletal maturation, and on predictions of adult stature must be monitored carefully.

Accurate measurement of the skeletal maturity of the knee would assist the surgical management of children with legs of unequal length. It is reasonable to expect that the effects of surgically induced epiphyseal fusion, performed to prevent the metaphyseal elongation of the femur or tibia, could be predicted better from the

maturity of the knee than from the maturity of the
hand-wrist.

Accurate skeletal ages of the knee would assist
the management of children with scoliosis, kyphosis or
lordosis because the timing of orthopedic surgery is
dependent, in part, on measures of skeletal maturity.
In addition, assessments of skeletal maturity of known
validity and accuracy would assist the analysis of
possible disassociations between the rates of skeletal
elongation and skeletal maturation during malnutrition,
illness, pubescence, "catch-up growth" and when the
blood supply to all, or part, of the skeleton is
abnormal, e.g., arteriovenous anastomoses, congenital
heart disease. Assessments of skeletal maturity are
used by many orthodontists to assist selection for
treatment, the choice of timing of treatment and to
provide better estimates of the future response to
treatment.

Anthropometric data are used to recognize and
grade malnutrition and to assess the effectiveness of
intervention programs in which supplementary foods are
provided (Brožek, 1956; Jelliffe, 1966; Jackson, 1966;
Malcolm, 1970; Roche and Falkner, 1974). Usually, the
effects of such intervention are considered favorable
if there is "catch-up growth" (Patton and Gardner, 1962;
Prader et al., 1963; Powell et al., 1967). However,
"catch-up growth" in stature is favorable only in the
absence of excessive acceleration of skeletal maturation
which would reduce the potential for growth in stature.
"Catch-up growth" should be analyzed by comparing
increments during biological age intervals. The best
biological ages for this purpose are valid, accurate
skeletal ages.

Other Possible Measures of Biological Age

The best estimate of biological age, a priori, is
chronological age. When an alternative measure, such
as skeletal age is used, differences between the
chronological and skeletal ages will be found in many

children. In these children, the bones are not estimating chronological ages accurately because they are
either more or less mature than is usual.

Skeletal maturity assessments can be made during
wider age ranges than other available measures of
biological age. For example, age in relation to
menarche or peak height velocity (the midpoint of the
year with the largest stature increment during pubescence) are applicable only to children who are near
the end of growth and, of course, age in relation to
menarche is limited to girls. The usefulness of age
in relation to peak height velocity is limited also
because it is applicable only to individuals for whom
there are long term serial growth data.

Changes in body shape occur during growth.
Perhaps the most obvious alterations are the pubertal
increases in the shoulder widths of boys and the hip
widths of girls. However, these and other measures of
general body shape differ widely among those who are
clearly adult. If these shape changes were used in a
biological age scale, some adults would be rated as
incompletely mature. Many systems for grading
secondary sex characters have been described. These
can provide useful biological ages only during the
chronological age ranges when they discriminate among
individuals, that is, about 9 to 16 years.

The level of dental development can be rated also,
either approximately by counting the number of teeth
erupted, or more accurately, by assessing the degree of
formation of the crown and root of each tooth (Sandler,
1944; Gleiser and Hunt, 1955; Garn et al., 1956;
Falkner, 1957; Fanning, 1961; Roche et al., 1964;
Demirjian and Goldstein, 1972; Demirjian et al., 1973).
The latter method is applicable over a wide age range
but it requires specialized radiographic equipment and
training. There are difficulties in using the level of
dental maturation as a biological age that is meaningful for the whole organism. All other biological age
scales show that girls are more advanced than boys

within chronological age groups but there are no significant sex differences in the timing of deciduous dental development (Doering and Allen, 1942; Robinow et al., 1942; Meredith, 1946; Roche et al., 1964). Furthermore, the correlation coefficients between dental development and either stature or skeletal age are almost zero in preschool children (Robinow et al., 1942). The permanent teeth, however, erupt earlier in girls than in boys (Clements et al., 1953; Kihlberg and Koski, 1954; Lee et al., 1965; Carlos and Gittelsohn, 1965); these sex differences vary among teeth (Hurme, 1949; Clements et al., 1953).

Skeletal age has been used more commonly than other measures of biological age because it has real meaning in regard to physical growth and development. There are significant positive correlations between skeletal age and the maturity levels of the reproductive system (Shuttleworth, 1938; Simmons and Greulich, 1943; Nicholson and Hanley, 1953; Hewitt and Acheson, 1961; Maresh, 1971). In addition, it is correlated significantly with body size (Wallis, 1931; Low et al., 1964), body shape (Acheson and Dupertius, 1957; Hunt et al., 1958; Hewitt and Acheson, 1961), the percentage of adult stature achieved (Simmons, 1944; Bayley and Pinneau, 1952), body composition (Jones, 1949; Maresh, 1961; Cheek et al., 1970) and the timing of peak height velocity and menarche (Maresh, 1971). Despite the general significance of skeletal age, if there is a need to determine the level of maturity of another body system, the maturity level of that system should be assessed directly and not inferred from skeletal age.

The Nature of Skeletal Maturation

A wealth of detail has been reported concerning the cellular and biochemical processes responsible for skeletal elongation but there is little corresponding knowledge concerning skeletal maturation. Some reports do not distinguish between elongation and maturation of the skeleton.

It is usual to consider that skeletal maturation
begins when the rudiments of bones can be recognized
in the embryo and that maturation is complete when
skeletal form and function become comparatively stable
in young adulthood. During this process, specialized
cells increase in number and their biochemical mechanisms become more complex. The present review is
applicable to most bones but specific examples relate
to the bones that form the knee joint.

    Histological changes. A long bone begins to
mature when some embryonic connective tissue condenses
to form a model (Gardner, 1963). In the early models
of most long bones, the parts that represent the future
diaphyses (shafts) are small, relative to the epiphyses,
although the junctions between these parts cannot be
identified with precision (Olivier and Pineau, 1959).
Gradually, the connective tissue model is replaced by
cartilage; this occurs first in the central part of
each model (Gardner, 1971). The surrounding connective tissue becomes a well defined layer called the
perichondrium. The inner zone of the perichondrium
contains cells that can mature into chondrocytes or
osteocytes; the outer zone differentiates to fibrous
tissue. These cartilaginous models resemble the shapes
of the bones they precede (Lewis, 1902; Hesser, 1926)
but adjacent models are joined by connective tissue at
the sites of future joints; joint cavities form later
(Gardner, 1971). These models enlarge by apposition
from the perichondrium, from the connective tissue
surrounding their ends, and by interstitial growth due
to the division of chondrocytes (Gardner, 1971).

    The centrally placed chondrocytes hypertrophy and
vacuolize at about the sixth prenatal week (Ham, 1969;
Gardner, 1971; Figure 1-A). This area calcifies (Niven
and Robison, 1934; Fell and Robison, 1934) and it
becomes visible radiographically when it is large enough.
This is the first stage of maturation that can be
observed in a radiograph. The area occupied by hypertrophic chondrocytes and calcified cartilage enlarges
rapidly and it extends along the cartilaginous model
(Figure 1-B).

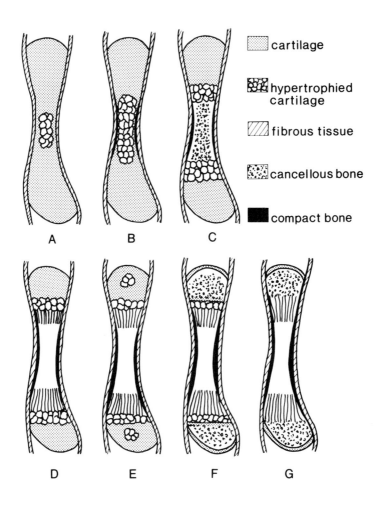

cartilage

hypertrophied cartilage

fibrous tissue

cancellous bone

compact bone

A   B   C

D   E   F   G

Figure 1. A diagram of the maturation of a long bone in which the length of the bone has been kept constant. The approximate age scale is: A, 6th prenatal week; B, 7th prenatal week; C, 12th prenatal week; D, 16th prenatal week to 2 years; E, 2 to 6 years; F, 6 to 16 years and G, adulthood. The clear area in D-G represents the marrow cavity.

Ossification begins when a collar of bone forms deep to the perichondrium around the central part of the cartilaginous model (Figure 1-B). Soon after this, ossification also begins by replacement of calcified cartilage centrally in the model where cartilage first formed (Rambaud and Renault, 1864; Gray et al., 1957; Brunk and Sköld, 1962; Gardner, 1971; Figure 1-C). In some bones, particularly vertebral bodies, the areas of calcified cartilage may be large and easily visible radiographically before ossification occurs (Hadley, 1956). The only convincing radiographic evidence that bone is present is the recognition of trabeculae; these may not be seen for a considerable period after the center becomes visible radiographically.

Endochondral ossification occurs in areas of cartilage where the chondrocytes have hypertrophied, the matrix has calcified and blood vessels, connective tissue cells and osteoblasts are present (Ham, 1969). These ossified areas extend along the cartilaginous model at similar rates both centrally (endochondral) and on the surface of the model (subperiosteal). Endochondral and subperiosteal ossification cannot be distinguished radiographically.

The areas of endochondral and subperiosteal ossification extend until they reach the levels of the future epiphyseal zones (epiphyseo-diaphyseal junctions) at each end of the model close to term (Felts, 1954; Figure 1-D). Before this occurs, resorption in the central part of the ossified area results in the formation of a small marrow cavity but this cannot be recognized radiographically until it is considerably larger. Radiographically visible changes occur in the shape of the end of the diaphysis (metaphysis) (Pyle and Hoerr, 1969) but the ossified area does not extend, in continuity, (epiphyseal fusion) beyond the epiphyseal zones at the knee, until about 16 years in boys and 14 years in girls (Pyle and Hoerr, 1969).

A most important stage of skeletal maturation occurs when an epiphyseal center of ossification forms within the cartilage at the distal end of the femur,

and the proximal ends of the tibia and fibula. This is
shown diagramatically in Figure 1-E. The histological
changes associated with endochondral ossification are
the same whether this occurs centrally in the model
or in the epiphyseal cartilages near each end of the
diaphysis (Gardner, 1971). The ossified area in each
epiphyseal cartilage enlarges more rapidly than the
cartilage and, within a few years, almost all the
cartilage is replaced, except for that in contact with
the end of the diaphysis (epiphyseal zone cartilage)
and on the articular surface (Figure 1-F).

At first, each epiphyseal ossification center
enlarges rapidly in all directions. Early, each center
is spherical and appears circular on a radiograph.
Later, it enlarges more rapidly in some directions
than others as its shape gradually approximates that
of the whole epiphyseal cartilage (Todd, 1930a; Pyle
et al., 1961; Gardner, 1971). This enlargement occurs
by the apposition of bone to each aspect of the center
except where it is in contact with the cartilage of the
epiphyseal zone (Payton, 1933; Siegling, 1941).

The transverse layer of epiphyseal zone cartilage
remains between the diaphysis and the ossified
epiphysis after most of the epiphyseal cartilage has
been replaced by bone. The chondrocytes in this zone
hypertrophy and vacuolize and the cartilage calcifies
preparatory to replacement by bone. These histological
changes are the same as those that occurred earlier
during ossification in the central part of the cartilage model. The changes are more regular in the
epiphyseal zone where there is a columnar arrangement
of chondrocytes and a corresponding orientation of
matrix and blood vessels. Together with the end of
the metaphysis, this layer is important in diaphyseal
elongation and also in the radiographic assessment of
maturity. The undulating shape of the layer may help
to prevent shearing through the zone of hypertrophic
cartilage cells (Johnson, 1966).

The aspect of the epiphyseal ossification center
in contact with the epiphyseal zone increases in cross-
sectional area more rapidly than either the end of the
diaphysis or the epiphyseal zone cartilage. The ratio
between the width of the ossified epiphysis and the
width of the metaphysis is important in the assessment
of skeletal maturation (Murray et al., 1971) despite
problems when it is used in some pathological states
(Acheson, 1966). There are three mechanisms by which
the epiphyseal zone cartilage increases in width:
proliferation in the deep layer of the cartilaginous
epiphysis, proliferation in the margin of the epiphyseal zone, and hypertrophy of chondrocytes within the
epiphyseal zone (Heřt, 1972).

The adjacent margins of the epiphyseal ossification center and the diaphysis gradually become
parallel. The associated radiographic changes are used
to assess skeletal maturity. Later, the diaphyseal
aspect of the epiphyseal center is covered by a thin
densely radio-opaque layer of bone (terminal plate)
which is used as a maturity indicator. The changes
that occur as the end of the diaphysis (metaphysis) is
progressively transformed and relocated during elongation to a more central position (Lacroix, 1951; Enlow,
1962) cannot be graded radiographically.

As adult levels of maturity are approached, a
thin undulating layer of bone covers the end of the
metaphysis and separates this from the calcified
cartilage of the epiphyseal zone (Moss and Noback,
1958; Silberberg and Silberberg, 1961). This layer
and the adjoining calcified cartilage cause a single
densely radio-opaque line that is used in assessment
(Park, 1954).

The final phase in the maturation of the long
bones of the knee joint is bony fusion of the epiphyses
to the diaphyses. Bony fusion appears to be completed
first in the central part of the zone (Stevenson,
1924; Todd, 1930; McKern and Stewart, 1957) despite
some opposite views (Haines and Mohuiddin, 1959, 1962).
Consequently, there is a period during which

ossification is incomplete in the peripheral part of
the epiphyseal zone cartilage causing a radiographically visible groove on the surface of the bone. The
transverse densely radio-opaque layer of bone that
joins the epiphysis to the metaphysis is resorbed after
fusion is complete but this resorption may be delayed
for a long period (Paterson, 1929; Sahay, 1941).
After fusion occurs, the articular cartilage is the
sole remnant of the cartilaginous model and the bone
is adult in maturity (Figure 1-G).

Many corresponding stages occur during the
maturation of the patella. A major difference is that
this bone does not develop epiphyseal ossification
centers or epiphyseal zones. The patella develops
first as a condensation of embryonic connective tissue.
Calcification occurs in this connective tissue and the
cartilaginous model that is formed resembles the future
bone in shape. This cartilaginous model articulates
with the femur; its other surfaces are covered by a
well-defined perichondrium. Ossification begins in
the cartilaginous model of the patella with the same
histological processes as those described for endochondral ossification of long bones and for the
ossification of epiphyseal centers. At first, the
ossified area expands rapidly in all directions;
later growth is more rapid in some directions than
others as the shape changes to match gradually that
of an adult patella (Gardner, 1971).

Radiographic Changes. Studies before the introduction of radiography drew attention to many macro-
scopic differences between the skeletons of children
and adults. These cross-sectional studies, using
dissection and histological techniques, were limited
to postmortem material. Knowledge of skeletal maturation increased rapidly with the application of
radiography. Only a few studies, selected from a very
large literature, will be mentioned.

Rotch (1908) described 13 stages in the development of the hand-wrist. Later, stages of carpal
maturation (Bardeen, 1921) and of epiphyseo-diaphyseal

fusion were described (Pryor, 1925; Hellman, 1928).
These workers did not develop systems for assessing
skeletal maturity but their studies led to the elabo-
ration of the Todd (1937) and Greulich-Pyle (1950,
1959) methods of assessment for the hand-wrist, the
atlas of Pyle and Hoerr (1955, 1969) for the assessment
of the knee and that of Hoerr, Pyle and Francis (1962)
for the foot-ankle.

    The radiographic appearances used to assess
skeletal maturity are known as "maturity indicators."
Each "indicator" that is useful in the assessment of
skeletal maturity must be present during the maturation
of every child (Pyle and Hoerr, 1969). Because of
limitations in the schedule of examinations, however,
there may be some or many children in whom a particular
indicator is not observed. By definition, these indicators appear in a fixed sequence for each bone (Todd,
1937; Pyle et al., 1948; Greulich, 1954; Pyle and
Hoerr, 1955; Greulich and Pyle, 1959; Tanner, 1962;
Acheson, 1966). This concept was stressed in Todd's
(1937) statement: "The sequence of maturity determi-
nators or symbols is always the same no matter what the
stock, parentage, economic standing, stature, weight or
health of the child."

    If Todd's statement were true, Tanner et al.
(1962, 1972) would not have needed to describe alternative criteria for maturity stages. In fact, the
sequence is not fixed for an area (Pryor, 1907; Todd,
1937; Abbott et al., 1950; Garn and Rohmann, 1960;
Hewitt and Acheson, 1961; Garn et al., 1966). This is
clear from the variations in developmental level that
occur between the bones of individuals (Pyle et al.,
1948; Greulich and Pyle, 1959; Poznanski et al., 1971;
Roche et al., 1974) and from variations in the order of
onset of ossification (Robinow, 1942; Kelly and
Reynolds, 1947; Garn and Rohmann, 1960; Christ, 1961;
Acheson, 1966; Yarbrough et al., 1973). These differences may be, but are not always, associated with ill
health (Sontag and Lipford, 1943; Garn et al., 1961;
Acheson, 1966). Differences in sequence occur also
between parts of a bone; this has been described for

the distal end of the femur and the proximal end of
the tibia (Roche and French, 1970).

Maturity indicators are based on the presence or
relative radiodensity of areas of calcification or
ossification. These differences in radiodensity
reflect the three-dimensional shapes of calcified or
ossified areas. The changes in contour, as bones
become more mature, reflect differences in the rates
of bone apposition at various bone surfaces. Parts of
the surfaces of these areas (especially the dense
cortex of bone) that are approximately parallel to the
central axis of the radiographic beam, cause dense
white zones on a radiograph. If these zones are long
and very narrow, they are referred to as "radio-
opaque lines."

Radiographs used for the assessment of skeletal
age must be taken under standardized conditions because
the radiographic appearance of bone outlines and radio-
opaque zones or lines is dependent on the inclination
of the radiographic beam. As will be noted later
(pp. 63-65), there were variations in positioning among
the radiographs used in the present study but it was
demonstrated that the substitutions made for standard
anteroposterior knee radiographs were justified.

The radiographic features that indicate maturity
provide information about the level of maturity in a
particular bone at the time the radiograph was taken.
If many serial radiographs are available for an individual, the duration of each indicator (or grade of
an indicator) can be determined, thus showing how long
the bone apparently remained at the same maturity
level. Information concerning the duration of an
indicator is potentially useful in developing a scoring
system because indicators that last a long time are
less informative than brief ones (Healy and Goldstein,
in press; Goldstein, personal communication, 1975).
Because the schedule of serial radiographs is always
related to chronological age rather than the inception
of maturity indicators, because there are "missed
visits" in all long term serial studies of children

and because the computational problems would be very
large, attempts have not been made to utilize this
property of indicators.

Many maturity indicators for the knee joint have
been described by Pyle and Hoerr (1969). The recognition and subjective grading of these is the basis of
the atlas method for assessing the skeletal maturity
of the knee. Their book includes 31 standards for the
maturity of the knee from birth to adulthood. Each of
these has two skeletal age equivalents--one for boys
and one for girls. These equivalents are expressed in
years and months of skeletal age. The standards show
the "central tendencies"* of maturity for children with
chronological ages matching the skeletal ages assigned
to the standards. When the atlas method is applied,
a radiograph is compared with these standards until
a standard is found that matches the radiograph in
maturity level, as determined from maturity indicators.
The skeletal age recorded for the radiograph is that
of the standard it matches. On occasions, it is
desirable to interpolate between standards or to apply
the procedure to individual bones. In the latter case,
bone-specific skeletal ages are recorded in years and
months. The accuracy of the method, whether applied
to an area or a bone is not known.

Scale of Maturity

The scale applied in the assessment of skeletal
maturity, using the atlas of Pyle and Hoerr (1969) is
based on the reasonable assumption that skeletal
maturity is absent at conception and that all individuals reach the same level of complete maturity in
young adulthood. The end point of this skeletal
maturity scale is the completion of epiphyseo-diaphyseal

---

* "Central tendencies" is used because Pyle and Hoerr
  (1969) did not select according to strict statistical
  criteria. Their "standards" are close to modes or
  medians.

fusion in bones with epiphyses and the attainment of adult shape in the patella.

By these premises, each individual achieves the same amount of maturation between conception and adulthood, although individuals differ in their rates of maturation. In practice, the origin of the scale is the onset of ossification in postnatal centers, as observed radiographically. Bones that develop epiphyseal ossification centers cannot be assessed reliably before this stage (Roche et al., 1970). Similarly, irregular bones, that do not develop epiphyses, such as the patella, cannot be assessed until they are visible radiographically.

When the atlas of Pyle and Hoerr (1969) is used to assess the knee, both anteroposterior and lateral radiographs are employed and either overall (area) or bone-specific skeletal ages are recorded. It is likely that the way in which these bone-specific ages for the knee are combined will alter the area skeletal ages that are assigned, as occurs for the hand-wrist (Roche and Johnson, 1969). In addition, it is possible to assess the medial and lateral condyles of both the femur and tibia separately (Roche and French, 1970) but the accuracy of such assessments is doubtful.

As stated earlier, the "standards" in the Pyle and Hoerr atlas represent the central tendencies of skeletal maturity levels in healthy children grouped by chronological age. The skeletal age levels, in years or months, assigned to these standards by the authors match the chronological age levels in their standardizing group. For example, the standard that matched the central tendency for girls aged nine years, in the group they studied, has been assigned a female equivalent skeletal age of nine years.

Two qualifications are necessary. The bones in the standards do, in fact, differ in maturity levels although this is not made clear in the Pyle and Hoerr atlas, as was done in the atlas of Greulich and Pyle (1959) for the hand-wrist. This makes the atlas

matching process less accurate, unless bone-specific
skeletal ages are recorded (Acheson et al., 1963;
Roche et al., 1970). If bone-specific assessments are
made, differences between bones will be found commonly
and the atlas of Pyle and Hoerr (1969) does not
describe how these bone-specific skeletal ages should
be combined. Secondly, the "standards" were derived
from a group of white children of very high socioeconomic status living in Cleveland, Ohio and enrolled
in the Brush Foundation Study. Although these
children were born between 1917 and 1942, and some
secular changes might be expected, skeletal maturity
standards for the hand-wrist (included in the Greulich-
Pyle atlas) are markedly in advance of the mean levels
of maturity in a national probability sample of United
States children (Roche et al., 1974, and in press).
The "standards" of Pyle and Hoerr (1969) for the knee
were derived from the same Brush Foundation children.
It is reasonable to assume that these standards, also,
are in advance of the mean levels for a truly representative sample of the present United States
population.

The Pyle and Hoerr (1969) skeletal maturity scales
for the knee are divided into years and months of
skeletal age but these intervals are not known to be
equivalent to each other. The scales are ordinal and
they do not provide a measurement of skeletal maturity
but allow a maturation level to be assigned to a radiograph relative to pictorial standards. Like other
ordinal scales, they permit rank ordering--in this
case, in regard to the level of skeletal maturity.

Typically, girls achieve adult levels of skeletal
maturity at younger chronological ages than do boys.
Therefore, more maturation occurs during a female
skeletal age year than during a male skeletal age year.
Furthermore, because individual bones differ in the
average chronological ages at which they reach adult
maturity levels (Roche et al., 1974), the percentage
of adult maturity achieved per skeletal age year
differs among bones.

A boy with a skeletal age of two years is more
mature than a boy with a skeletal age of one year but
he may not be twice as mature. The amount of maturation between one and two years may not be equivalent
to that between birth and one year. Because of the
way in which the Pyle and Hoerr scale was constructed,
these skeletal age "units" (years, months) are not
necessarily equivalent to each other. However,
because all boys mature until they reach the same
adult level of maturity, it can be concluded that all
boys at the same skeletal maturity level have achieved
the same percentage of adult maturity, although the
actual percentage is unknown. This is the major advantage of the scale of skeletal maturity. By contrast,
many physical characteristics of children, e.g.,
weight are recorded using a ratio scale, i.e., they
admit only to multiplicative transformations because
they have a fixed zero point. These scales allow the
calculation of ratios between measures, e.g., a boy
weighing 70 kg is twice as heavy as a boy weighing
35 kg. Because adults differ in weight, two boys, each
weighing 60 kg, may not have achieved the same percentages of their adult weights.

The major alternative scale to a series of atlas
standards with skeletal age equivalents is based on
assigning "scores," or numbers, to bones depending on
their levels of maturity. This system, first known
as the Oxford method, was introduced by Acheson (1954)
who applied it to the hand-wrist and knee in preschool
children. Later it was extended to the hip and the
age range was increased (Acheson and Dupertuis, 1957;
Hewitt and Acheson, 1961). Originally, the hand-wrist
scores were modified by differential weighting among
bones in order that the mean values for the group of
preschool children studied by Acheson should have a
straight line relationship to chronological age. The
unweighted knee scores for the group were related to
chronological age in a rectilinear fashion.

The Oxford method has advantages. The obligation
to score bones separately and to recognize precise
indicators forces the assessor to examine individual

bones with care. This is necessary because commonly
(or perhaps always) the bones of an area differ in
maturity level. Consequently, the Oxford method led
to increases in objectivity but the manner of scoring
is unsatisfactory because the inferences that can be
made from summing across bone scores obtained in this
way are limited (Lord, 1953).

Tanner and his colleagues (1962, 1971, 1972,
1975) improved and extended the Oxford method. The
Tanner-Whitehouse method, as it is generally known, is
applicable to the hand-wrist throughout the whole range
of maturity. It makes use of approximately 8 maturity
indicators for each of 20 selected hand-wrist bones.
In this selection, the bones of the second and fourth
"rays"* were omitted, which is unwise because their
skeletal maturity levels are correlated highly with
those of corresponding bones in the other "rays"
(Roche et al., 1970; Sproul and Peritz, 1971). If an
underlying trait is to be rated by indirect means, it
is preferable to use indicators that are highly correlated (Wilks, 1938; Wainer, 1975). It would be better
to adopt a more generous attitude and also select
bones that have high communality indices with all
other bones of the area, as has been suggested (Garn
and Rohmann, 1959; Garn et al., 1964). An assessment
method restricted to highly representative bones
would fail to utilize potentially important information available from bones that tend to be divergent.
The maturity status of the latter may be a sensitive
indicator of environmental effects.

The original Tanner-Whitehouse method (TW-I) was
modified in 1972; the present description refers to
the revised method (TW-II). The scores assigned to
the stages of each bone were derived as follows.
It was assumed that the observed stages of each bone

* A ray of the hand consists of a metacarpal and its
  associated phalanges, e.g., metacarpal II, proximal
  phalanx II, middle phalanx II and distal phalanx II.

of the individual all reflect the same underlying
quantity, skeletal maturity. Scores were assigned
so that the disparity between the scores for the
individual, summed over all individuals in the
standardizing group, is minimal. The mathematical
method is described in Healy and Goldstein (in press)
and is one of a general class of scaling procedures.
The method requires at least two points of the scale
to be fixed. These have been determined by requiring
the average of all the initial stages to be zero and
the average of all the final stages to be 100, thus
defining a scale running from zero to 100 (Healy and
Goldstein, in press; Goldstein, personal communication,
1975).

The contribution of each bone to the total score
was weighted on an arbitrary biological basis. The
aim of minimizing disagreement between bones for the
whole group has some validity but the extent of its
implementation must be determined subjectively. At
the extreme, the same score would be assigned to each
bone; there would be no disagreement and little
information. This aim implies that the bones of the
hand-wrist of an individual are normally at the same
level of maturity, which is close to Todd's (1937)
concept of the evenly maturing skeleton. This concept
receives strong support (Roche et al., 1975) from a
recent analysis of the structure of bone-specific
skeletal ages in the hand-wrist, foot-ankle and knee
assessed by the atlas method (Greulich and Pyle, 1959;
Hoerr et al., 1962; Pyle and Hoerr, 1969).

In the TW-II method, three skeletal ages are
obtained: an age based on all the 20 bones graded, one
based on the carpals only and one based on the radius,
ulna and selected short bones. Half the total score
is derived from the carpals by assigning a large
weighting to each of these bones.

The Tanner-Whitehouse method assumes a fixed
sequence of maturity indicators for each bone, but
some stages have multiple criteria. A particular
stage is allocated to a bone only after the first

possible should be used and that all the useful
relevant information should be obtained from each
radiograph. The present choice was an anteroposterior view of the knee joint.

Assessment of one joint area, rather than
bilateral corresponding areas, is acceptable
biologically. Lateral asymmetry in the onset of
ossification of diaphyses is rare in the hand (Noback
and Robertson, 1951; Meyer and O'Rahilly, 1958) and
unusual in the foot (Noback and Robertson, 1951;
Meyer and O'Rahilly, 1958; Kraus, 1961) and pelvis
(Francis, 1951). Pryor (1907) and Sawtell (1929)
expressed opinions that unilateral presence of an
ossified center was unusual during childhood; this is
in agreement with the findings of other investigators
(Spencer, 1891; Menees and Holly, 1932; Elgenmark,
1946; Tarleton et al., 1960). There are, however,
contrary data, partly from Pryor's own study (1936)
of two sets of quadruplets but mainly from reasonably
large groups of children, that such lateral differences are common (Long and Caldwell, 1911; Flecker,
1932; Torgensen, 1951; Christ, 1961; Roche, 1963).
All the workers, who have found lateral differences
in the number of centers ossified, or the particular
bones ossified, agree that these differences are
small (usually one center in an individual) and of no
practical importance.

Early workers established that there are no real
lateral differences between the sums of carpal areas
(Baldwin et al., 1928), the maximum diameters of
radial epiphyses (Sawtell, 1929) and radial indices
based on epiphyseal and metaphyseal widths (Sawtell,
1929). In addition, many later studies have shown
only small non-significant systematic lateral differences in skeletal maturity levels (Rotch, 1908;
Bardeen, 1921; Sawtell, 1929; Pryor, 1936; Flory,
1936; Schmid and Halden, 1949; Dedick and Caffey,
1953; Dreizen et al., 1957; Baer and Durkatz, 1957;
Greulich and Pyle, 1959; Roche, 1963). However,
others have reported the unusual occurrence of lateral
differences in skeletal maturity as large as 6 months

(Dreizen et al., 1957; Christ, 1961) or even 12 months (Borovanský and Hněvkovský, 1929) in normal children. Despite the large differences that are observed rarely, there is no doubt that the reported findings justify the now almost universal decision to assess only one side of the skeleton.

Why the Knee?

The hand-wrist is assessed more frequently than other areas, partly because it was the first area for which atlases of standards were available (Howard, 1928; Flory, 1936; Todd, 1937; Greulich and Pyle, 1950). Furthermore, the standards in the popular Greulich and Pyle atlas for the hand-wrist are much clearer than those of Pyle and Hoerr (1969) for the knee or those of Hoerr, Pyle and Francis (1962) for the foot-ankle. Some prefer the hand-wrist because many bones are present in a relatively small area but there is no doubt that many of these bones, e.g., proximal phalanges, provide redundant information (Hayman, 1959; Tanner et al., 1962; Clarke and Hayman, 1962; Clarke and Degutis, 1962; Roche, 1970; Sproul and Peritz, 1971; Roche et al., 1974).

The hand-wrist is easier to position for radiography than the knee joint but positioning of the latter for an anteroposterior view is not difficult. It is, however, not so easy to obtain direct lateral views of the knee. A more important matter is that there are long age ranges (particularly 11-15 years in boys and 9-13.5 years in girls) during which the hand-wrist provides little information concerning changes in the level of skeletal maturity (Sauvegrain et al., 1962).

Problems occur in assessments of the hand-wrist, using the Greulich-Pyle atlas, towards the end of maturation because some bones in this area, e.g., distal phalanges, reach adult levels at about 15 years in boys and 13.5 years in girls (Todd, 1930; Pyle

et al., 1961; Garn et al., 1961a; Hansman, 1962). After
this occurs, only the designation "adult," and not a
skeletal age expressed in years, can be applied to
them. A mean area skeletal age for the hand-wrist
cannot be derived from a set of bone-specific
"skeletal ages" some of which are "adult." Nevertheless, a median can be calculated if less than half
the bones are "adult."

The principles involved in determining whether
the carpals should be included when the hand-wrist is
assessed are relevant to the development of a maturity
scale for the knee. Many agree that the carpals are
markedly variable in rates and patterns of maturation
(Baldwin et al., 1928; Wallis, 1931; Todd, 1937;
Francis and Werle, 1939; Bayer and Newell, 1940;
O'Rahilly, 1953; Hewitt et al., 1955; Driezen et al.,
1958, 1959; Garn and Rohmann, 1959, 1960). Some have
concluded that they should not be assessed because
their rates of maturation are so variable (Todd, 1937;
Johnston and Jahina, 1965; Acheson, 1966).

This variability in rate would be an advantage
if it assisted meaningful discrimination among
individuals. Evidence has not been presented, however,
that the levels of maturity of the carpal bones in
normal children provide useful information over and
above that provided by the maturity levels of the
other bones of the hand-wrist. The frequency with
which the patterns of maturation of carpal bones differ
among individuals makes it difficult to apply the
single set of standards provided by Greulich and Pyle
for each sex. In the RWT method, all useful indicators
have been retained even if the morphology of the area
being graded were markedly variable. When this was
the case, a range of shapes at the same maturity level
has been provided in Chapter IV.

The area to be assessed should be determined
partly by the reason for the assessment. For example,
if a measure of skeletal maturity is required to
estimate the potentials for elongation at the knee
joints of an anisomelic child, the knee joints should

be assessed. When an assessment of skeletal maturity
is requested by a pediatrician for a child whose stature
deviates from the mean, the knee area is preferable to
the hand-wrist. The knee is an important site of growth
in stature and it can provide a slightly more accurate
estimate of the potential for growth in stature than
the hand-wrist (Roche et al., 1974), even when assessed
using the atlas of Pyle and Hoerr (1969).

In addition to the above, the knee was chosen for
a practical reason. When this attempt to devise a new
method was commenced, the methodology that had to be
used had not been developed. Consequently, there were
many unsuccessful exploratory efforts, particularly in
the early phases of the work. The process of designing
satisfactory criteria for indicators and determining
the usefulness of possible indicators was very difficult
and time consuming, although only three bones were
involved. The statistical combination of data from the
three bones assessed (femur, tibia and fibula) required
complex procedures. As a result of the experience
gained, it is now feasible, however, to extend the
investigation and to develop a corresponding method for
the hand-wrist. This would have been impractical earlier.

Current Methods for Assessing the Knee

Although a method for assessing the knee in
preschool children was described by Acheson (1954), the
only method in current use is that of Pyle and Hoerr
(1955, 1969). Despite its defects, the atlas of Pyle
and Hoerr provided the first complete published method
for assessing the knee. Earlier, Todd (1930a) described
many radiographic changes that occur during the maturation of the knee joint. In addition, prior to 1935,
he prepared a tentative atlas of knee maturity
"standards." These standards were selected from
radiographs of children enrolled in The Brush Foundation
Study. It was from these, and later radiographs of the
same children, that Pyle and Hoerr (1969) selected
their maturity standards for the knee. This set of
Todd standards for the knee was not published but was

tested and used by several investigators in the United
States (Bayley, 1943; Macy, 1946; Kelly and Macy, 1958).

The method of Pyle and Hoerr is based on 31 standards derived from a large group of Cleveland children
examined between 1929 and 1942 who were very much above
average in socioeconomic status. As stated earlier,
there is little doubt that the maturity levels in the
Pyle and Hoerr atlas are too high for the present total
United States population.

The first step in the selection of the Pyle and
Hoerr standards was to work backwards, from the oldest
to the youngest, through the serial radiographs for
individuals, to identify maturity indicators and to
establish approximate ages for their appearance in each
sex. Some indicators used in the Pyle and Hoerr atlas
are unsatisfactory because they are based on comparisons
between bones, e.g., "The tibial metaphysis is about
90 percent as wide as the femoral metaphysis"(p.42).
Each bone should be assessed independently; each indicator should refer to one bone only.

Pyle and Hoerr had available Todd's unpublished
set of maturity standards for the knee. In constructing their scale, they used about 400 sets of radiographs
that extended to 10 years and about 250 sets for the
period from 10 years to maturity. The early part of
the scale was completed using radiographs taken at The
Harvard School of Public Health because the earliest
radiographs had been taken at 3 months in The Brush
Foundation Study. It is likely that the use of radiographs from two populations caused some irregularity in
the Pyle and Hoerr scale of maturity because the Harvard
group tended to be retarded in hand-wrist skeletal
maturity compared with the Brush Foundation children
(Bayley, 1962). Probably,a similar difference would be
present between the two groups in the rates of maturation at the knee joint.

When Pyle and Hoerr considered the listing of
maturity indicators complete for a bone, they commenced
the selection of standard radiographs. This was done,

for each sex separately, by choosing the radiograph that represented best the central tendency of maturity for each bone (femur, tibia, fibula and patella) when 100 radiographs, at each six months of age, were arrayed in order of maturity level. Radiographs were chosen as standards on the basis of the <u>most mature bone in each radiograph</u>. For example, the standard radiograph for boys aged 7 years was "assessed," bone by bone, by comparison with other radiographs that had been placed in order of maturity. These bone-specific assessments for the standard radiograph may have been:

femur	6.8	years
tibia	7.0	years
fibula	6.9	years
patella	6.7	years.

However, the skeletal age equivalent of the most mature bone (femur, 7.0 years) would have been assigned to the whole area if this radiograph had been used as a standard in the Pyle and Hoerr atlas. This procedure must have led to the systematic choice of standards that were more advanced than the central tendency of the Cleveland group but the extent of the differences introduced by this procedure are unknown.

This selection procedure reflects the opinion of Todd (1937) and others (Pyle et al., 1948; Macy and Kelly, 1957) who considered all bones would be at the same maturity level in a healthy child, but that illnesses retarded the maturation of some bones more than others and thus cause dysharmonic maturation. According to this view, the most advanced bone represents the unhindered normal level for the child. Standards were selected on the basis of what should have been-- not what was. Nevertheless, an assessor applying the method attempts to estimate the actual level of maturity. The effect of this method of selection would have been reduced had Pyle and Hoerr instructed assessors to assign the skeletal age of the most mature bone in each radiograph to the whole knee area.

Later Pyle and Hoerr combined the two sex-specific series of standards to a single unisex series; male and female skeletal age equivalents were assigned to

each standard plate. For example, their Plate 8 shows
a maturity level to which a male skeletal age of
18 months and a female skeletal age of 15 months are
assigned.

Pyle and Hoerr assumed that the stages of skeletal
maturation, and their sequence, are the same in each
sex. Proof that the sequence is the same has not been
available. Sex dependent patterns in the carpus (Garn
et al., 1967; Thompson et al., 1973) and, more certainly, in the hip, have been described (Hewitt and
Acheson, 1961).

There may be sex-related differences in the knee
also. There are differences between males and females
in the order of ossification of centers near the knee
(Garn et al., 1966) and the patterns of age-associated
changes in the ratio medial condyle height/lateral
condyle height for the femur differ between the sexes.
After 6 years, the means for this ratio remain essen-
tially constant in boys but they decrease markedly in
girls (Scheller, 1960). While the components of such
a ratio reflect size, the ratio itself is a measure of
shape and is relevant to skeletal maturity status.
Furthermore, in the present study, it was shown that
the adductor tubercle became universal in boys but not
girls.* Garn et al. (1971) claimed "... with the
details of the maturational scheme far from identical
in males and females it does not seem appropriate to
use the same pictorial standards with separate sex-
equivalents, at least for more systematic scientific
comparisons." Chapter VII contains some findings from
the present study that are relevant to this matter.

The atlases from the Cleveland School (Todd,
1937; Greulich and Pyle, 1950, 1959; Pyle and Hoerr,
1955, 1969; Hoerr et al., 1962) are based on the theory
that the maturity indicators within a bone, and within

---

* It is not retained among the final indicators for
  boys because the change in prevalence with age was
  too slow for it to be useful.

an area, develop in a regular sequence. However, studies of the sequence of maturity indicators among bones have not been reported in detail except in regard to the onset of ossification and epiphyseo-diaphyseal fusion (Moss and Noback, 1958; Garn and Rohmann, 1960; Garn et al., 1961a; Yarbrough et al., 1973). Both these stages show differences in sequence within areas but not to extents that invalidate the atlas method.

When the Pyle and Hoerr atlas is used, specific skeletal ages cannot be assigned to two groups of bones in some radiographs: bones that are not radio-opaque can be rated only as "less than x years;" those that are adult can be rated only as "more than y years," where, for each sex, x and y respectively are the mean ages at which the bone becomes radio-opaque and adult. These ratings cannot be used to calculate means.

If mean skeletal ages were derived only from the remaining bones, some illogical changes could occur in serial area skeletal ages for individuals. For example, if the proximal epiphysis of the fibula were markedly retarded in onset of ossification, it would be omitted in the calculation of a mean skeletal age until it is ossified. When it did ossify, the low skeletal age assigned to it could reduce the area skeletal age for the knee. Some have attempted to circumvent this dif- ficulty (e.g., Lee, 1971) but a satisfactory method has not been reported.

In the Pyle and Hoerr atlas, practically no attention is given to the range of shapes and appear- ances that may be present at the same maturity level. It is not easy to be sure that the same maturity levels correspond to various shapes of a particular bone. In the present RWT system for the knee, when appropriate, a range of shapes is illustrated for each grade of the maturity indicators. The low prevalence of reversals (retrograde changes in apparent maturity levels with increasing chronological age) in serial data from indi- viduals for these indicators showed that the assignment of the same indicator grade to these ranges of shapes was justified.

In the Pyle and Hoerr atlas, however, only a
single standard plate is provided for the whole knee
joint in both sexes at any one maturity level. In fact,
some differences between successive standards apparently are due not to changes in maturity but to individual differences in the extents to which "maturity
indicators" are developed in children at the same
maturity level. For example, the standards for skeletal
ages 108 through 144 months in boys show increasing
development of the intercondylar tubercles of the tibia
but these tubercles are much less developed in the
standards for skeletal ages 153 through 165 months.
The failure to give sufficient attention to individual
variation may stem from the attitude expressed by Hoerr,
Pyle and Francis (1962). In their atlas for the assessment of the foot-ankle, they state that one should
"discount the variant bone from the calculation of
skeletal age."

The Pyle and Hoerr atlas does not provide information about the ranges of levels of skeletal maturity
among normal children. Most importantly, it does not
provide a description of the method by which it should
be used. Assessors probably vary widely in the ways
they apply it, as occurs with the Greulich and Pyle
atlas (Roche and Johnson, 1969). Some investigators
subjectively combine the maturity levels of individual
bones to obtain an area skeletal age (Pyle et al., 1959)
while others have used the mean or other combinations
of these ages as the area skeletal age (Roche, 1967;
Roche and Johnson, 1969; Roche et al., 1974).

CHAPTER II

SUMMARY OF LITERATURE

RELATING TO THE MATURATION OF THE KNEE

In this section, as the title implies, the intention is to summarize the previous literature. A critical review is not presented because this could not be done effectively without including many findings from the present study. The present account will be restricted to the changes visible in an anteroposterior radiograph after birth. Consideration will not be given to the patella, which cannot be seen clearly in this view.

Although the atlas of Pyle and Hoerr (1955, 1969) gives little attention to normal variations in shape and has other defects, it is the major source of information concerning the maturation of the knee joint. Unless noted otherwise, the account in this summary is based on their text. All the ages given in the summary are for boys; the corresponding ages for girls would be younger. Table I includes the approximate sex differences in the ages at which particular maturity levels of the knee are reached. As can be seen in the table, a single radiograph assessed against the unisex standards in the Pyle and Hoerr atlas as having a skeletal age of 52 months, if a radiograph of a boy, would have a skeletal age of 36 months if it were a radiograph of a girl. Christ (1929) and Schmid and Halden (1949) have claimed, somewhat surprisingly and incorrectly, that there are no sex differences in the rates of maturation at the knee.

TABLE I

Central Tendencies for
Ages (Skeletal Age,
Months, Male) at Which
Boys and Girls Reach
the Same Levels of
Maturity in the Knee
(Based on Roche, 1968)
and the Standards in
the Atlas of Pyle and
Hoerr (1969)

Boys			Girls
5	equivalent	to	4
11	"	"	9
15	"	"	12
23	"	"	19
35	"	"	23
41	"	"	26
46	"	"	30
52	"	"	36
58	"	"	40
70	"	"	54
82	"	"	62
91	"	"	71
103	"	"	79
115	"	"	87
127	"	"	93
139	"	"	103
156	"	"	120
163	"	"	127
175	"	"	143
199	"	"	169

Mention should be made also of the work of Takahashi (1956) who recorded the incidence of some "intermediate maturity indicators"* in 300 Japanese children studied cross-sectionally at ages from 7 to 19 years (Table II). While he did report the ages at which these indicators were present in 50 percent of the children studied, Takahashi did not attempt to develop a method of assessment based on these findings.

Femur--Distal End

At birth, there is a small indentation in the distal margin of the metaphysis near the midline (Figure 2); soon this indentation becomes distinct and relatively deep (Pyle and Hoerr, 1969). At one month, it is about half as wide as the metaphysis and it is almost two-thirds as wide at 6 months. This proportion is about the same at 12 months despite marked flaring of the metaphysis (Figure 3) between birth and one year (Ingalls, 1927; Pyle and Hoerr, 1969).

Ossification occurs in the epiphysis about 2 weeks before birth (Figure 2; Adair and Scammon, 1921; Pryor, 1923; Menees and Holly, 1932; Hill, 1939; Gray and Gardner, 1950; Hartley, 1957). At birth, the ossified area is oval, with smooth margins and with its long axis at right angles to that of the shaft (Hartley, 1957; Pyle and Hoerr, 1969). By one month, it has become ovoid, its lateral end is the larger and its vertical height is equal to about half its width. Earlier reports (Fick, 1901; Schmid and Halden, 1949) that it does not become ovoid until about 6 months are incorrect.

* An intermediate "maturity indicator" is a radio-graphically visible feature that assists the assessment of skeletal maturity and that appears between the onset of ossification and the completion of maturation (epiphyseo-diaphyseal fusion in a long or short bone).

TABLE II

Ages (Years) at Which "Maturity Indicators" Are Present
in 50 Percent of Children Studied Cross-sectionally
(from Takahashi, 1956)

Stage	Boys	Girls
FEMUR		
III. The proximal end of the lateral epicondyle is sharp. Both epicondyles are angular.	7.1	----
IV. Proximal ends of both epicondyles are sharper. The epiphysis caps the diaphysis.	10.6	----
V. Capping has progressed. The epiphysis is as wide as the diaphysis. The epiphyseal zone is narrower.	13.5	12.2
VI. The epiphyseal zone is narrower.	15.3	13.7
VII. Epiphyseo-diaphyseal fusion is incomplete.	17.1	15.0
VIII. Fusion is complete but the line of fusion is still visible.	18.0	17.0
TIBIA		
III. The intercondylar notch is deeper. The lateral margin of the lateral condyle begins to flatten and form square corners with the articular and metaphyseal margins.	8.6	----
IV. The medial margin forms square corners with the articular and metaphyseal margins.	10.0	9.0

TABLE II (continued)

Stage	Boys	Girls
V. The epiphysis caps the metaphysis.	13.2	10.7
VI. Capping has progressed and the epiphysis is as wide as the metaphysis.	15.0	12.7
VII. The epiphyseal zone is thinner.	15.7	14.3
VIII. Epiphyseo-diaphyseal fusion has begun.	16.7	15.7
IX. Epiphyseo-diaphyseal fusion is just completed. The line of fusion is visible.	17.4	16.3
X. The line of fusion is obliterated or faint.	----	18.2

FIBULA

Stage	Boys	Girls
V. The styloid process begins to form.	11.0	----
VI. The styloid process is better differentiated and the medial margin begins to flatten.	13.1	11.6
VII. The lateral margin extends beyond the metaphysis and the styloid process is larger.	14.4	13.0
VIII. The epiphyseal zone is thinner.	15.7	13.6
IX. Epiphyseo-diaphyseal fusion is incomplete.	16.8	15.7
X. Epiphyseo-diaphyseal fusion is complete.	18.2	17.2

There has been much interest in the ratio
epiphyseal width/metaphyseal width. Assessments of
skeletal maturity are based almost entirely on the
shapes of bones. Some elements of these shapes can be
summarized effectively using ratios between linear
measurements. These ratios can provide useful information about skeletal maturity levels although each
measurement separately is unable to do so because each
indicates size, not shape. The data of Scheller (1960),
on which Table III is based, supersede the reports of
Fick (1901), Ludloff (1903) and Cohn (1922) who studied
very small groups of children. In addition, data from
so long ago is suspect with regard to its applicability
to the children and youth of today. The mean values
reported by Scheller are in close agreement with those
of Mossberg (1949) which are included in Table IV.
Both sets of data indicate rapid changes and rather
large sex differences until about five years. Later,
the changes are much less rapid and the sex differences
are slight. These reported data indicate that this
ratio could be a useful indicator of skeletal maturity
at young ages.

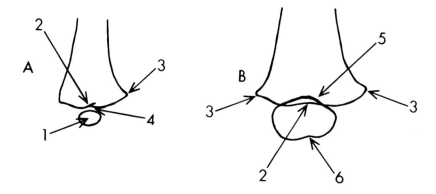

Figure 2. Femur. A, birth; B, 9 months. 1 = epiphysis,
2 = indentation in metaphysis, 3 = flaring of metaphysis,
4 = epiphyseal zone, 5 = terminal plate and 6 = indentation in epiphysis (intercondylar notch).

Calcified strands and areas in the epiphyseal cartilage, beyond the ossified area, occur between 2 and 4 years (Christ, 1929; Sontag and Pyle, 1941; Ribbing, 1944; Scheller, 1960). This is known as disseminated calcification (Figure 3). It may be associated with rapid growth of the epiphyseal carti- lage or with a thick zone of calcification around a rapidly growing center of ossification in the epiphysis (Sontag and Pyle, 1941; Pyle and Hoerr, 1969).

Roughness of the non-articular margins of the femoral condyles may have a similar biological basis. This roughness is common, being more marked on the medial than the lateral margin in the large group of

TABLE   III

Means for the Distal Femoral
Ratio Epiphyseal Width/
Metaphyseal Width
(based on Scheller, 1960)

Age	Boys		Girls	
(years)	N	Mean	N	Mean
1.5	3	62	9	80
2.5	16	76	18	91
3.5	19	87	15	95
4.5	20	92	9	98
5.5	20	96	15	100
6.5	29	98	11	103
7.5	27	100	14	103
8.5	36	102	23	104
9.5	37	103	40	106
10.5	44	104	51	107
11.5	59	106	61	107
12.5	62	107	52	108
13.5	52	108	44	107
14.5	41	109	25	108

radiographs studied by Scheller (1960). A similar
distribution of disseminated calcification was reported
by Sontag and Pyle (1941). However, using a much
smaller group of radiographs and combining roughness of
the condylar margins with disseminated calcification,
Caffey, Samuel, Royer and Morales (1958) concluded that
these appearances, considered together, were more
common on the lateral margin.

Disseminated calcification has been described by
Pyle and Hoerr (1969) as a skeletal maturity indicator
although it is absent in almost all children by 6 years.
For this reason, it cannot be a useful indicator unless
serial data are available. If disseminated calcification is absent from a single radiograph that is to be
assessed, there is no way of knowing whether it has not
yet developed or whether it was present earlier.

TABLE   IV

Means for the Distal Femoral
Ratio Epiphyseal Width/
Metaphyseal Width
(based on Mossberg, 1949)

Age	Boys		Girls	
(years)	N	Mean	N	Mean
2	39	70	39	77
4	36	87	29	96
6	39	97	25	101
8	38	102	27	104
10	40	105	36	107
12	38	107	35	108
14	38	110	35	110
16	34	109	20	110
18	19	109	7	104

At 6 months, the epiphysis is curved reciprocally with the wide shallow indentation in the end of the metaphysis, except for flaring of the ends of the epiphyseal zone. The lateral end of the epiphysis is blunter than the medial and a terminal plate (Figure 2) is visible on its metaphyseal margin. Pyle and Hoerr (1969) state that, at 9 months, the epiphyseal zone has the thickness that is characteristic for most of the growing period, but later they claim this zone has become thinner (2 years), as is clearly the case.

At 9 months, the distal margin of the epiphysis is slightly indented near the midline; this is the first radiographic indication of the future intercondylar notch (Figure 4). The epiphysis extends medially and laterally slightly beyond the metaphyseal indentation. At 2 years, the intercondylar notch is relatively narrower, being 25 to 33 percent as wide as the epiphysis. The lateral non-articular margin of the epiphysis (Figure 4) is flattened slightly and its medial end is more rounded than previously. At 2.5 years, the epiphysis is wider; only a small part of the metaphysis extends laterally beyond it whereas almost one third of the medial part of the metaphysis extends beyond the epiphysis. At 3 years, the ends of the epiphyseal zone do not flare as markedly as previously.

Early, the lateral condyle is taller than the medial (Figures 2 and 4); later this is reversed at ages variously reported as 2, 3.5 and 4.75 years

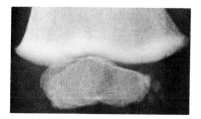

Figure 3. An example of disseminated calcification of the distal end of the femur.

(Ludloff, 1903; Scheller, 1960; Pyle and Hoerr, 1959).
Considering the sample sizes available to these authors
at the critical ages, the latter figure, from Pyle and
Hoerr, must be regarded as the most reliable.

The medial condyle is wider than the lateral at all
ages (Scheller, 1960); not only after 6 years, as reported
by Ludloff (1903), who studied a very small group of
radiographs. In fact, the ratio medial condyle width/
lateral condyle width tends to decrease with age but these
changes are only slight (Scheller, 1960; Table V).

At 4 years, the intercondylar notch is well marked.
At 4.5 years, corners form at the junctions of the
terminal plate with the non-articular margins of the
epiphysis (Figures 4 and 5) and both the condylar articular surfaces become more rounded.

At 5 years, the medial half of the metaphyseal margin
of the epiphysis is concave proximally. There is recip-
rocal curving between the epiphysis and the metaphysis

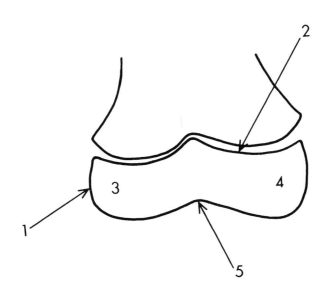

Figure 4. Femur--4 years. 1 = lateral non-articular
margin, 2 = concavity of medial part of metaphyseal
margin of epiphysis, 3 = lateral condyle, 4 = medial
condyle and 5 = intercondylar notch.

except for some widening of the ends of the epiphyseal zone. The lateral end of this zone may appear double because of its complex curvature in three dimensions.

At 6 years, the intercondylar notch is deeper. The epiphysis is not as wide as the metaphysis and its lateral margin continues smoothly into the articular surface (Figure 5). The lateral and medial epicondyles begin to form and sharp corners develop between the medial margin and the metaphyseal and articular margins (Figure 5).

TABLE V

Means for the Distal
Femoral Ratio
Medial Condyle Width/
Lateral Condyle Width
(based on Scheller, 1960)

Age	Boys		Girls	
(years)	N	Mean	N	Mean
1.5	3	126	9	122
2.5	16	111	18	119
3.5	19	117	15	119
4.5	20	115	9	120
5.5	20	116	15	118
6.5	29	114	11	121
7.5	27	117	14	115
8.5	36	115	23	114
9.5	37	113	40	113
10.5	44	113	51	108
11.5	59	112	61	109
12.5	62	112	52	104
13.5	52	109	44	104
14.5	41	112	25	101

At 7 years, the metaphyseal and lateral margins of the epiphysis meet at a sharp angle (Figure 5), indicating ossification of the epiphyseal part of the lateral epicondyle. The lateral articular surface begins to flatten near the intercondylar notch.

At 8 years, the junction between the metaphyseal and the lateral margins of the epiphysis begins to project proximally; this area is slightly less dense than the rest of the lateral condyle. The lateral and articular surfaces of the lateral condyle join at a blunt angle. The articular margin of the medial condyle is rounded; its medial non-articular margin is rough and variable in radiodensity.

At 9 years, a low protuberance (Figure 6) divides the lateral margin of the lateral condyle to two flat surfaces. Popliteus arises, in part, from the distal of these surfaces. The medial margin of the medial

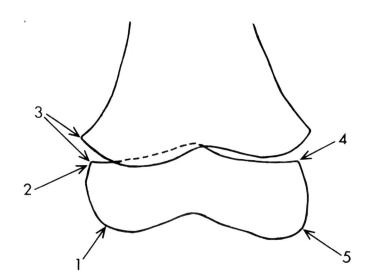

Figure 5. Femur--7 years. 1 = junction of lateral and articular surfaces, 2 = junction of lateral and metaphyseal margins, 3 = lateral epicondyle, 4 = medial epicondyle and 5 = junction of medial and articular margins.

condyle is smooth and is joined to the articular surface
by a rounded curve. The epiphyseal part of the medial
epicondyle is more uniformly calcified. The terminal
plate curves into the medial and lateral epicondyles
and the medial end of the epiphysis begins to cap the
metaphysis (Figure 6).

At 10 years, a thin radio-opaque line bounds a
relatively radiolucent oval facet just inside the
lateral margin of the metaphysis. This facet indicates
an area of attachment of the lateral head of gastrocnemius (Figure 6). There is some capping of the
metaphysis by the epiphysis medially and laterally
(Figure 6). The medial epicondyle is now a rounded
prominence distal to the beak-like projection at the
medial end of the metaphyseal margin. The non-articular
and articular margins of the lateral condyle join at a
distinct corner. An almost vertical radio-opaque line
inside the lateral margin of the epiphysis marks its
postero-lateral edge (Figure 6).

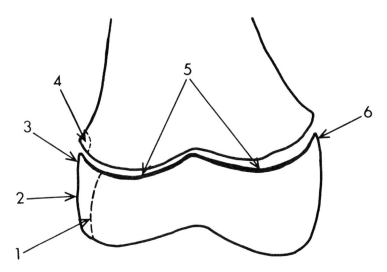

Figure 6. Femur--9 years. 1 = posterolateral edge of
lateral condyle, 2 = protuberance on lateral condyle,
3 = lateral capping of metaphysis by epiphysis,
4 = radiolucent facet (lateral head of gastrocnemius),
5 = terminal plate and 6 = medial capping of metaphysis
by epiphysis.

At 11 years, the adductor tubercle (Figure 7) is
a sharp projection from the medial end of the metaphysis; the medial epicondyle is distal to this. An
indistinct thin line is present within the medial part
of the epiphysis; probably this line is due to the
posteromedial edge (Figure 7).

At 12 years, the pointed tip of the epiphyseal
part of the lateral epicondyle has a minute, relatively
radiolucent triangular area. The lateral part of the
epiphyseal zone is thinner. The terminal plate curves
near the adductor tubercle. A transverse trabecular
pattern alongside the patella (Figure 7) radiates
towards the medial condyle where the trabeculae
are vertical.

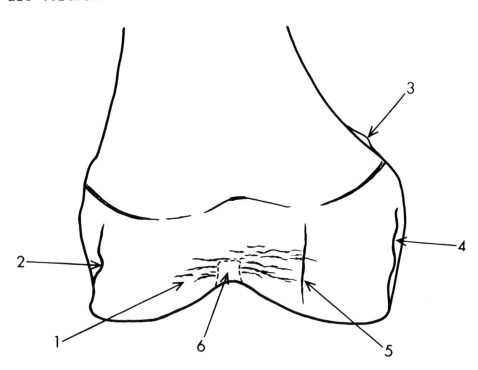

Figure 7. Femur--16 years. 1 = transverse trabecular
pattern, 2 = notch for popliteus, 3 = adductor tubercle,
4 = posteromedial edge of epiphysis, 5 = medial margin
of intercondylar fossa, and 6 = relatively translucent
area.

At about 12.5 years, an angle begins to form
between the articular and medial margins of the medial
condyle. At 13 years, the central part of the epiphyseal zone is fuzzy but the terminal plate remains.
A vertical line indicates the medial margin of the
intercondylar fossa (Figure 7). The beak-shaped corner
of the epiphysis at the junction between the metaphyseal
and lateral margins marks part of the attachment of
gastrocnemius. The articular and most of the non-
articular surfaces of the medial condyle are flat and
there is a definite rounded angle between these margins.

At 14 years, the metaphysis has become more radio-
opaque; the epiphyseal zone is thinner centrally.
There is a rectangular region of relative radiolucency
proximal to the intercondylar notch (Figure 7). The
line due to the postero-lateral margin of the lateral
condyle has become definitely notched for the tendon
of popliteus (Figure 7). The junction between the
articular and lateral surfaces of the lateral condyle
is almost rectangular and the epiphysis caps the
metaphysis closely.

At 14.5 years, the epiphyseal zone is indistinct
along its length; this precedes epiphyseo-diaphyseal
fusion. The facets on the lateral non-articular margin
are outlined clearly. The central part of the articular margin of the lateral condyle is more radio-opaque
than the remainder. The angles dividing the articular
and non-articular surfaces of the epiphysis are sharper
now than they will be later.

At 16 years, some traces of the epiphyseal line
remain but the terminal plate of the epiphysis is still
thick. The lateral margin of the lateral condyle is
relatively straight. The medial articular surface is
less rounded. A line that is concave laterally runs
proximally from the angle between the medial margin and
the articular surface. At 17 years, the epiphyseal
zone is much thinner but fusion is incomplete.

At 17 years, epiphyseo-diaphyseal fusion is complete. This age, taken from the standards of Pyle and

Hoerr (1969), is close to those reported by Cohn (1922), Todd (1930), Flecker (1942) and Vandervael (1952). A slightly younger age (16.6 years) has been reported for Denver boys by Hansman (1962). A thick radio-opaque line at the level of the epiphyseal zone usually indicates that fusion occurred recently. After fusion, the trabecular pattern becomes similar in the former epiphysis and metaphysis and the angles between the articular and non-articular surfaces are smooth.

The difficulties of identifying incomplete fusion or recently complete fusion have been emphasized by several workers (Stevenson, 1924; Todd, 1930, 1937; Ray et al., 1950; Joss et al., 1963). The present investigation has shown that satisfactory criteria can be established and that the classification of fusion need not be delayed until there is "entire disappearance of the epiphyseal plate" (Flecker, 1942). However, as will be shown later, a knee radiograph provides insufficient information for an accurate estimate of skeletal age when adult levels of maturity are approached.

Tibia--Proximal End

In full term infants, the epiphysis (Figure 8) begins to ossify about one week before birth (Adair and Scammon, 1921; Paterson, 1929; Menees and Holly, 1932; Hill, 1939; Gray and Gardner, 1950), occasionally from two centers that soon fuse (Köhler and Zimmer, 1956). At birth, the ossified area is elliptical with a smooth margin. It grows in width more rapidly than in height; consequently, the width is about twice the height at one month. The central part of the metaphysis (Figure 8) is flattened at this time. At 3 months, the epiphysis is symmetrically elliptical. The epiphyseal zone (Figure 8) is uniform in thickness centrally but it widens at each end.

Reported data relating to the ratio epiphyseal width/metaphyseal width for the tibia are in Tables VI

and VII. These ratios are higher in girls than in boys
at all ages through 20 years (Mossberg, 1949; Scheller,
1960). The increases in the means are small after
10 years; consequently, this indicator could be useful
at young ages only. In passing, it should be emphasized that this ratio can be a valid indicator of
maturity although the individual measures that are
combined in the ratio indicate size and tend to be
larger in boys than girls within chronological age
groups (Stuart et al.,1940).

At 6 months, the adjacent metaphyseal and epiphyseal margins are reciprocally flattened over an area
that is about two-thirds as wide as the end of the
metaphysis. There is an incomplete terminal plate
(Figure 8) on the metaphyseal margin of the epiphysis
that appears first on the medial part. At 9 months,
the epiphyseal zone has the thickness that is characteristic for most of the growing period.

The lateral and medial parts of the articular
surface of the epiphysis begin to flatten obliquely
(Figure 8); this is the first stage in the formation
of the intercondylar eminence (Figure 9). Scheller
(1960) considers this occurs during the first year but

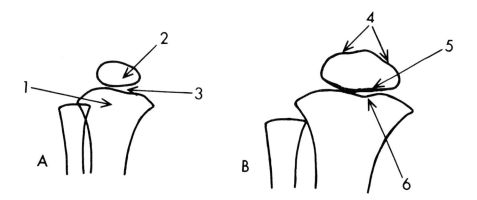

Figure 8. Tibia. A, birth; B, 15 months. 1 = metaphysis, 2 = epiphysis, 3 = epiphyseal zone, 4 = lateral
and medial articular surfaces, 5 = terminal plate and
6 = indentation in metaphysis.

Pyle and Hoerr (1969) first describe it at 1.2 years.
The latter figure should be accepted because Scheller
had too small a group of boys in this age range (N = 8)
for his judgment to be reliable. The metaphysis is
indented near the midline (Figure 8) where a cartilaginous tongue extends distally from the epiphysis.

At 1.5 years, the lateral condyle is narrower than
the medial (Figure 8) and the medial margin is pointed.
The medial part of the articular surface is flat and
there is a radio-opaque line on its margin (Figure 9)
which precedes the medial articular facet. The epiphyseal zone widens at each end. At 1.9 years, the medial
part of the articular surface is slightly concave.

At 2 years, the non-articular margins of the
epiphysis (Figure 9) are taller and its metaphyseal

TABLE   VI

Means for the Proximal Tibial
Ratio Epiphyseal Width/
Metaphyseal Width
(based on Mossberg, 1949)

Age	Boys		Girls	
(years)	N	Mean	N	Mean
2	39	69.5	39	72.0
4	36	81.8	29	90.6
6	39	94.3	25	104.7
8	38	104.8	27	110.4
10	40	110.7	36	113.3
12	38	113.6	35	114.6
14	38	115.6	36	117.6
16	36	116.6	33	115.9
18	40	115.9	38	110.0
20	36	112.4	38	118.2

margin is relatively opaque. The epiphyseal zone is narrow and more uniform in thickness.

At 2.5 years, the lateral half of the articular surface is slightly concave (Figure 9) and the medial non-articular margin is no longer pointed. A radio-opaque line extends across the intercondylar eminence (Figure 10) which no longer has a pointed apex.

The onset of ossification in the tibial tuberosity (Figure 9) is visible as a small midline extension from the metaphyseal margin of the epiphysis, opposite an indentation in the metaphysis. At first, this extension is triangular but it becomes approximately rectangular at 8 to 11 years. A separate center appears

TABLE VII

Means for the Proximal Tibial
Ratio Epiphyseal Width/
Metaphyseal Width
(based on Scheller, 1960)

Age	Boys		Girls	
(years)	N	Mean	N	Mean
1.5	--	--	9	75
2.5	16	75	18	83
3.5	19	77	15	88
4.5	20	85	9	95
5.5	20	93	15	104
6.5	29	97	11	110
7.5	27	103	14	109
8.5	36	107	23	111
9.5	37	110	40	113
10.5	44	111	51	114
11.5	59	113	61	115
12.5	62	114	52	116
13.5	52	115	44	116
14.5	41	115	25	116

near the distal margin of the extension at 9 to
10 years. This center forms in about 50 percent of
children. This center fuses with the proximal tibial
epiphysis at 13 to 14 years and with the shaft at
16 years. The additional center cannot be seen clearly
in an anteroposterior radiograph (Francis, 1940; Pyle
and Hoerr, 1955; Köhler and Zimmer, 1956).

At 3.5 years, the lateral end of the epiphyseal
zone flares more than the medial. The lateral condyle
is now the wider. The medial half of the articular
surface is outlined clearly and there may be disseminated calcification on the non-articular epiphyseal
margins (Figure 10). At 4 years, the intercondylar
tubercles are present. The medial margin is still
convex and the ends of the epiphyseal zone flare
slightly.

At 4.5 years, the base of the intercondylar
eminence is crossed by a thin radio-opaque line that is
placed anteriorly (Figure 10). The lateral part of

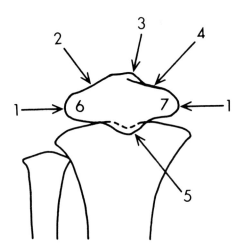

Figure 9. Tibia--2 years. 1 = lateral and medial
non-articular margins, 2 = lateral part of articular
surface, 3 = intercondylar eminence, 4 = radio-opaque
line on margin of medial condyle, 5 = tibial tuberosity,
6 = lateral condyle and 7 = medial condyle.

the articular surface is smooth and the medial part is
distinctly concave, as shown by the shape of the radio-
opaque line that crosses the bone and extends to the
non-articular margin (Figure 10). Tomographic studies
show that this line is due to the posterior margin of
the articular surface (Scheller, 1960), not the anterior
as has been claimed (Pyle and Hoerr, 1969). The terminal plate projects distally near the midline where
the tibial tuberosity extends from the margin of the
epiphysis.

At 5 years, the intercondylar eminence is a broad
plateau and the tips of the tubercles (Figure 10) are
outlined by relatively radio-opaque zones. Occasionally, the intercondylar eminence is sufficiently large
to obscure the tubercles. An angle is forming between
the articular surface and the lateral margin.

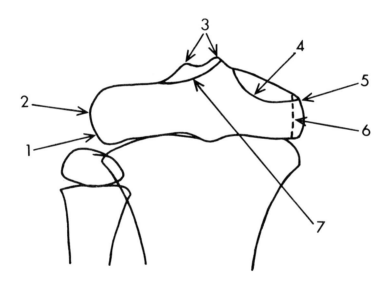

Figure 10. Tibia--7 years. 1 = site of tibio-fibular
joint, 2 = lateral non-articular margin, 3 = intercondylar tubercles, 4 = radio-opaque line across medial
condyle, 5 = junction of articular and non-articular
margins of medial condyle, 6 = posteromedial edge of
medial condyle and 7 = radio-opaque line across base of
intercondylar eminence.

At 6 years, the intercondylar tubercles are
rudimentary. The lateral non-articular margin is
flatter (Figure 10). The medial condyle is rectangular
with a distinct corner between its articular and non-
articular margins (Figure 10).

At 7 years, the tubercles are slightly higher than
the general level of the eminence. The lateral condyle
is becoming rectangular. The part of the medial condyle between the radio-opaque line and the articular
margin is now more radio-opaque. The lateral end of
the epiphyseal zone is the widest part. The tongue of
the epiphysis that projects across the epiphyseal zone
as part of the tibial tuberosity is acquiring a definite outline.

At 8 years, all the articular and non-articular
margins are flat except the lateral non-articular
margin, which is rough. Corners are forming where the
metaphyseal margin of the epiphysis joins its medial
and lateral margins (Figure 10). At 9 years, there is
a distinct notch between the intercondylar tubercles,
which are clearly outlined by thin radio-opaque lines.
The radio-opaque line across the medial condyle is
considerably distal to the margin.

At 10 years, the intercondylar eminence has
enlarged and its tubercles project considerably beyond
the concavities of the articular facets. The anterior
and posterior margins of the lateral articular facet
can be distinguished; the anterior is the denser and
the more concave. A thin radio-opaque line within the
medial edge of the epiphysis is probably due to the
postero-medial edge of the condyle (Figure 10). The
distal half of the lateral margin is flattened and
slopes medially, marking the site of the tibio-fibular
joint (Figure 10). Depressions for the semilunar
cartilages are present (Cohn, 1922).

At 11 years, the medial condyle is larger than the
lateral (Cohn, 1922). The terminal plate has extended
to the lateral side of the epiphysis. The central part

of the epiphyseal zone is fuzzy where the tibial
tuberosity crosses it.

At 12 years, the intercondylar eminence is tall
and the tubercles are relatively radiolucent, with their
surfaces marked by radio-opaque lines. Typically, the
tubercles are more pointed than previously.

At 13 years, the small indentation between the
intercondylar tubercles has a radio-opaque margin.
The sides of both condyles are taller than the central
parts of their articular surfaces. The ends of the
metaphysis are bevelled and the terminal plate caps
these areas (Figure 11). The lateral margin is straight
except for a slight indentation near its center in the
area of the tibio-fibular joint.

At 14 years, the anterior margin of the medial
articular surface is much more radio-opaque than the
adjacent bone. The terminal plate of the epiphysis caps

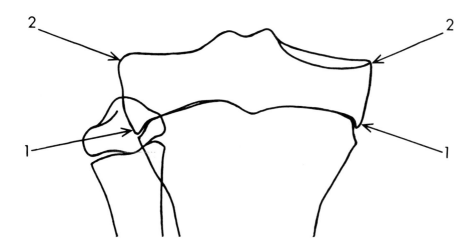

Figure 11. Tibia--15 years. 1 = capping of metaphysis
by epiphysis and 2 = junctions between articular and
non-articular surfaces.

the metaphysis closely and the metaphysis is more
radio-opaque.

At 14.5 years, the medial non-articular margin has
become taller and flatter. At 14.8 years, the terminal
plate is more radio-opaque, preceding epiphyseo-
diaphyseal fusion. The whole epiphyseal zone is
indistinct; it is thinner centrally and scarcely
enlarged at its ends. The angles at the junctions
between the articular and non-articular surfaces are
sharper now than they will be later (Figure 11).

At 15 years, the epiphyseal zone has become very
thin. At 15.5 years, there is some fusion centrally
and medially. At 17 years, a few small remnants of the
epiphyseal zone remain and fusion is complete at
18 years. There are rounded junctions between the
articular and non-articular surfaces and the medial
tubercle is higher than the lateral.

The age of fusion, as indicated in the Pyle and
Hoerr (1969) standards, is in general agreement with
the report of Flecker (1942) but is later than the ages
of 16.2 and 16.9 years reported by Garn et al. (1961a)
and Hansman (1962) respectively.

Fibula--Proximal End

The proximal epiphysis of the fibula (Figure 12)
ossifies at about 3.7 years (Pyle and Hoerr, 1969).
This is in close agreement with the findings of Garn,
Rohmann and Silverman (1967) but Hansman (1962)
reported a median age of 4.4 years. Each of these
studies was based on an adequate number of children.
Probably there were real differences between the groups
studied. There are corresponding differences between
the Denver and Fels groups in the ages at onset of
ossification in other bones and in pubertal events
(Maresh, 1972; Hansman, 1962; Garn et al., 1967; Roche,
unpublished data).

At 4.5 years, the epiphyseal zone (Figure 12) is straight and wide and there is slight disseminated calcification. The epiphyseal zone is narrower centrally than at its ends. At 6 years, there is a terminal plate along most of the metaphyseal margin (Figure 12). The epiphysis is dome shaped, reaching to the level of the epiphyseal zone of the tibia.

At 7 years, the part of the epiphysis near the medial margin is slightly more radio-opaque than the remainder (Figure 12). An articular facet will develop in this area at the level of the epiphyseal zone of the tibia. The medial margin is slightly indented at 8 years when the epiphysis is two-thirds as wide as the metaphysis (Cohn, 1922).

At 9 years, the tibio-fibular articular facet is forming just distal to the tibial epiphysis. There is a rounded junction between this facet and the proximal margin of the epiphysis. At 11 years, the styloid process begins to form (Figure 12). At 12 years, there is an indentation, marked by a radio-opaque line, in the articular margin lateral to the styloid process (Figure 12). At 13 years, a horizontal radio-opaque

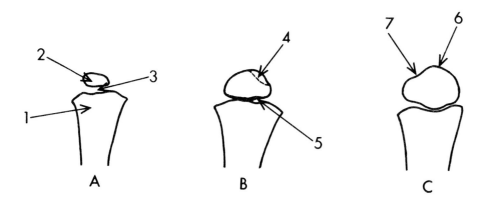

Figure 12. Fibula. A and B, 2-6 years; C, 13 years. 1 = metaphysis, 2 = epiphysis, 3 = epiphyseal zone, 4 = radio-opaque area for tibio-fibular joint, 5 = terminal plate, 6 = styloid process and 7 = indentation lateral to styloid process.

line crossing the epiphysis indicates the articular facet.

At 14 years, the epiphysis is as wide as the metaphysis. At 16.3 years, the epiphyseal zone is very thin; the articular facet and the indentation in the head of the fibula are almost complete. At 17 years, the epiphyseal line is extremely thin except its lateral part. The last area to fuse is on the antero-lateral aspect (McKern and Stewart, 1957).

At 18 years, fusion is complete. This is in general agreement with the findings of Flecker (1942), Vandervael (1952) and Hansman (1962) but Garn, Rohmann and Apfelbaum (1961a) reported a mean age for fusion of 17.2 years. As for the other bones of the knee joint, Stevenson (1924) and Todd (1931) incorrectly considered there was no sex difference in the timing of epiphyseal fusion.

CHAPTER III

MATERIAL AND METHODS

Children

Many aspects of the 279 boys and 273 girls studied
during the development of the new method have been
described previously (Sontag et al., 1958; Crandall,
1972). These children live in Southwestern Ohio and
were born between 1928 and 1972. Their homes are
within 30 miles of Yellow Springs, about 35 percent
living in cities of medium size (population 30,000-
60,000), about half in small towns (population 500-
5,000) and the remainder on farms. The educational
and occupational patterns for these three groups do
not follow the usual urban-rural differences. About
15 percent of the fathers are professionals or major
executives, 35 percent are businessmen, 35 percent are
tradesmen or white collar workers and the remaining
15 percent are skilled or semiskilled laborers. About
60 percent of the parents attended a year or more of
college and about 60 percent of them were born in Ohio.
In general, they were of middle socioeconomic level.
These children were enrolled in utero. Commencing in
1929, about 15 children joined the study each year.

The children were examined by a pediatrician at
each scheduled visit. Treatment was not provided but
parents were recommended to consult their family phy-
sician when appropriate. Some of the children had
clinical conditions that could have influenced the
rates or patterns of skeletal maturation. The incidence of these conditions was no greater than one would
expect in the general population. When the conditions

59

not be due to differences in radiographic or assessment techniques. The above hypothesis concerning a
secular trend was tested in two ways; firstly, by
calculating the correlation coefficients, within
selected chronological age groups, between skeletal
ages (RWT and Greulich-Pyle) and year of birth
(Table IX). If there were a positive secular trend,
i.e., maturation occurring more rapidly in recent years
than a few decades ago, one would expect statistically
significant correlation coefficients between year of
birth and the skeletal ages at particular chronological
ages. This analysis showed that, if any such trend were
present, it was slight and could be disregarded. A
second test was made by comparing maturity levels
between parents and children of the same sex when both
were at the same chronological age (Table X). The mean

TABLE X

Mean Relative Differences between
Parent-Offspring Pairs in Skeletal Age
(RWT, Knee in Years). + = Parent More Mature

| Chronological Age (years) | Difference | | | | | |
| | Father-Son | | | Mother-Daughter | | |
	N	Mean	s.d.	N	Mean	s.d.
6	25	-.33	1.16	33	-.16	1.17
7	24	-.15	1.36	35	+.21	1.10
8	23	+.40	1.14	32	+.23	1.40
9	25	+.29	1.32	29	+.08	1.35
10	21	+.12	1.45	19	-.35	1.28
11	17	+.16	1.32	20	-.95	1.52
12	14	+.24	1.89	21	-.14	1.00
13	8	+.04	1.36	17	-.15	0.98
14	9	+.17	0.75	17	-.32	1.15
15	8	-.93	0.59	19	-.62	1.71
16	8	-.02	0.51	10	-.57	1.48

differences between fathers and sons are generally
small and they differ in direction as various chronological age groups are considered. There is a tendency for the mothers to be less mature than their
daughters at the same chronological ages but this is
slight. The mean differences are overshadowed by the
large standard deviations of these differences in each
chronological age group for both the male and female
pairs.

     Comparisons were made between the ages at menarche
of mothers and daughters. Both members of each pair
were participants in the Fels Longitudinal Study. The
relevant information had been obtained by 6-monthly
enquiry at appropriate ages. The mean difference
(N = 23) was 0.03 years, with the mothers tending to
be later by this clearly insignificant amount.

     The anteroposterior non-screened radiographs that
were used were of three types:

     (i) knee (A in Table XI). The joint was extended
fully; the central ray was at the level of the joint
and at right angles to the long axis of the femur and
tibia. The tube-film distance was 91.4 cm. These
radiographs were suitable for grading all the final
indicators. Review of serial data and sets of radiographs showed that minor flexing of the knee joint, in
this or the other types of radiographs, did not affect
the grading of the final indicators.

     (ii) Standing leg (B in Table XI). These were
taken standing with a tube-film distance of 121.9 cm.
The central ray was directed midway between the two
knees. These radiographs were satisfactory for almost
all the final indicators.

     (iii) lower leg (C in Table XI). The radiographic
field included the knee and ankle joints. These were
taken standing or recumbent (tube-film distance 182.8 cm)
with the central ray at right angles to the long axis
of the tibia and at the level of its midpoint. The
image of the knee joint was slightly distorted in these

TABLE XI

Number of Radiographs Used in Scale Construction

Age	Boys				Girls			
	A	B	C	Total	A	B	C	Total
1 month	---	---	113	113	---	---	125	125
3 months	---	---	87	87	---	---	100	100
6 months	---	---	128	128	---	---	144	144
9 months	---	---	83	83	---	---	100	100
1.0 years	23	---	141	164	23	---	118	141
1.5 years	93	---	17	110	99	---	17	116
2.0 years	130	2	27	159	113	17	12	142
2.5 years	93	---	14	107	107	2	2	111
3.0 years	121	2	31	154	113	14	10	137
3.5 years	94	---	5	99	96	1	7	104
4.0 years	113	9	29	151	103	21	12	136
4.5 years	98	1	1	100	88	2	2	92
5.0 years	112	11	17	140	104	20	3	127
5.5 years	80	5	5	90	75	3	2	80
6.0 years	176	---	37	213	172	1	23	196
6.5 years	9	98	13	120	2	93	5	100
7.0 years	190	---	11	201	194	---	10	204
7.5 years	1	103	9	113	1	92	4	97
8.0 years	181	---	6	187	177	---	12	189
8.5 years	19	86	7	112	14	77	2	93
9.0 years	168	---	15	183	165	---	10	175
9.5 years	6	2	40	48	7	8	65	80
10.0 years	164	---	11	175	158	---	8	166
11.0 years	149	---	---	149	138	---	---	138
12.0 years	137	---	---	137	134	---	---	134
13.0 years	133	---	---	133	121	---	---	121
14.0 years	127	---	---	127	118	---	---	118
15.0 years	116	---	---	116	106	---	---	106
16.0 years	105	---	---	105	102	---	---	102
17.0 years	98	---	---	98	74	---	---	74
18.0 years	92	---	---	92	52	---	---	52
Totals	2828	319	847	3997	2656	351	793	3800

A = knee; B = standing leg; C = lower leg.

radiographs and they could be used for very few indicators. However, they were the only radiographs available from one to nine months.

The number of radiographs used to develop the new scale is shown in Table XI. If more than one of the three types of radiographs was available for a child at a particular age, only one was used. Knee radiographs were used in preference to others, not because of concern about differences in enlargement but about the effects of variations in radiographic positioning. If a knee radiograph was not available for a child at a particular age, a standing leg radiograph was substituted. If neither a knee nor a standing leg radiograph were available, a lower leg radiograph was used.

These substitutions were made only if the results of two test procedures showed they were justified. Firstly, for each indicator, comparisons were made of data from sets of radiographs of individuals taken at the same age with these three techniques. The findings from these comparisons were used to determine whether standing leg or lower leg radiographs could be substituted for knee radiographs when the latter were not available. Secondly, for each indicator within its associated age range, trials were made employing series of radiographs for individuals before radiographs other than knee radiographs were used. Substitutions were made only if the trials showed no reversals in the serial trends at ages when other types of radiographs were used. If the results of these surveys of sets of radiographs and of data from serial radiographs both showed that a substitution for knee radiographs could be made for a particular indicator during a defined age range, other radiographs were substituted and rated in the same way as knee radiographs.

The alterations in the tube-film distances for the knee and lower leg radiographs during the study were of little concern because, as expected, variations in enlargement did not alter the recording of indicators.

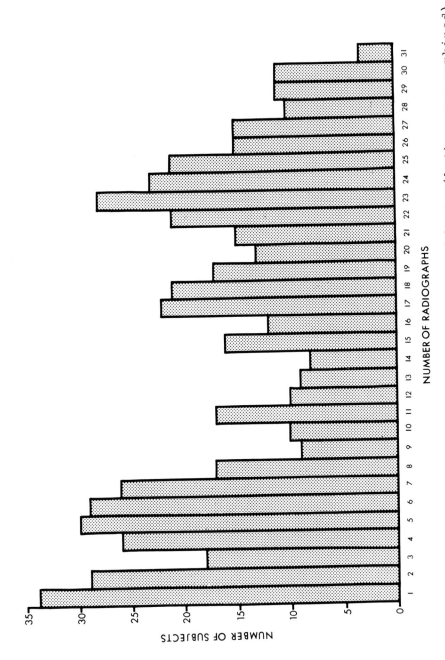

Figure 13. A histogram showing the numbers of subjects (both sexes combined) with particular numbers of serial radiographs.

The radiographs were taken at ages from one month to 18 years. Additional radiographs at older ages (20-26 years) were used to test the universality of late occurring indicators. The scheduled ages were 1, 3, 6 and 9 months, after which the examinations were 6-monthly to 10 years and then annual to 18 years. Further radiographs were taken biennially of many participants. The radiographs were taken at chronological ages that were very near the scheduled ages. The limits were ±1% of the chronological age except at 1 and 3 months when the limits were ±1 day and at later ages when the limits did not exceed ±25 days. For example, all radiographs of boys aged "10 years" were taken within 25 days of the tenth birthdays of these boys.

The number of radiographs utilized was 3997 for boys and 3800 for girls. As will be seen later (Chapter VII), some of these radiographs (particularly near the younger and older limits of the age range) did not provide sufficient information about maturity level to be useful. As stated earlier, these films had been taken of 279 boys and 273 girls. Consequently, there was a marked serial component in the radiographic data. The extent of this is shown in Figure 13.

Many lateral radiographs of the knee were available but these were not used. The aim was to develop an effective system of skeletal age assessment of the knee using a single anteroposterior radiograph, thus minimizing irradiation. Due to this exclusion, the patella was not included among the bones graded.

Methodology

Any system for determing skeletal maturity status from a radiograph must depend on the recognition of maturity indicators. Data derived from indicators can be transformed to a skeletal age equivalent by subjective comparison with atlas standards or by objectively weighting data from each indicator. The problems inherent in atlas comparisons have been considered

earlier (pp. 29-32). The aim of the present study was
to develop an alternative method based on the grading
and weighting of "useful" maturity indicators.

Maturity indicators are radiographically visible
features that undergo successive changes during the
maturation of a bone. Most are due to the replacement
of cartilage by bone; others are due to bone growth
at subperiosteal surfaces or bone resorption. These
mechanisms lead to changes in shape that are reflected
in radiographic outlines and dense radio-opaque lines
or areas.

Throughout the present study, emphasis was on these
"maturity indicators" because they provide all the
information a radiograph can supply for the assessment
of skeletal maturity. Necessarily, all methods are
based on them but their grading, weighting and combination are too subjective and unstructured in the atlas
method of Pyle and Hoerr (1955, 1969).

As stated by Garn (Roche, 1971), the real need is
to simplify assessments and to base them only on indicators known to be useful. The rationale of the
present investigation was to determine the usefulness
of each possible indicator and to describe those
selected completely and without ambiguity. The aim was
to design a method that would provide a measure of the
error of the estimate and in which the replicability
of assessments was not influenced by variant orders of
maturation among and within bones. It is considered
that these aims have been achieved.

Nine steps were taken to determine the usefulness
of the "maturity indicators" described in the literature. The procedure was developed using radiographs of
boys; later it was applied to the girls. This sequence
of boys first, girls later was appropriate because
skeletal maturation proceeds more slowly in boys than
in girls yet the scheduled ages for radiography were the
same in each sex.

The serial radiographs of the boys present, to
some extent, "slow motion" views of maturation compared
to those presented by the serial radiographs of the
girls. An additional factor leading to this choice was
the fact that some possible indicators, e.g., the adductor tubercle, reflect levels of muscular development and
were considered likely to be more conspicuous in boys
than girls. Neither of these factors was mandatory;
the alternative sequence of girls then boys could have
been adopted without difficulty.

The study was extended to girls after suitable
criteria had been determined for boys and useful indicators had been selected by the steps to be described.
The major purposes in this extension to girls were to
determine whether any of the indicators were sex-
limited, to define the age ranges during which they
should be assessed, and, of course, to obtain the data
needed for the preparation of a computer program for
the estimation of skeletal age in girls.

Step 1. Lists of possible indicators were compiled
from the literature, the most important sources being
Pyle and Hoerr (1955, 1969) and Scheller (1960). These
indicators were collated for each bone in the region of
the knee joint and they were placed in their approximate order of appearance.

Step 2. The descriptions of the indicators were
rewritten so that they would be applicable to the full
range of shapes likely to be present in radiographs of
normal children. As far as possible, the terminology
was standardized and made more correct anatomically.
Some of the terms used are defined in the glossary
(pp. x-xi).

Many descriptions of indicators in the literature
are too vague to be useful. For example, "the lateral
condyle (femur) is blocky" (Pyle and Hoerr, 1969, p.81).
This indicator was not tested because the shape of the
lateral condyle classed as "blocky" was reflected in

indicators relating to the shape of the articular and
non-articular margins of the condyle and the curvatures
of the junctions between them. Some other indicators
described in the literature were excluded because they
referred to more than one bone. For example, Pyle and
Hoerr (1969, p. 48) describe a stage when the tibial
epiphysis becomes as wide as the femoral epiphysis.
The tibia should be rated against group data for the
tibia, not the femur. Rating against the femur would
be appropriate only if one were sure that, within the
radiograph being assessed, the femur and tibia did not
differ in maturity level.

Step 3. Methods that are as objective as possible
were developed to grade particular indicators. In
general, an excessive number of possible grades was
tested for each indicator; later these were combined
as the need for this became clear during testing.

Necessarily some of the indicators tested were
assessed subjectively. For example, "the epiphyseal
portion of the lateral epicondyle has become a small
triangular area of lesser density" (Pyle and Hoerr,
1969, p. 85). The criteria for these indicators were
made as definite and as close to objective as possible.

Many indicators described in the literature are
based on the curvature of margins of radiographic
shadows, e.g., "the(medial tibial) condyle is rectangular, its articular facet is typically concave, and
a distinct osseous corner marks off the side of the
condyle from the articular facet" (Pyle and Hoerr, 1969,
p. 72). Subjective judgments of curvatures lack comparability and repeatability (as measured by interobserver
and intraobserver differences) especially if applied to
single, as opposed to serial, radiographs. These indicators were graded by fitting mathematically constructed
curves drawn on tracing plastic.* The curves were of
fixed length for each indicator and were either the

---

* Readily available from art supply houses (cellulose
acetate, matte transparent, .003" thick).

major or minor poles of ellipses (Table XII, Figure 14)
drawn using a drafting template.[*]

Some of the maturity indicators were ratios
between linear measurements. These can be used as
maturity indicators, if they meet the necessary criteria, although the separate measurements combined in
each ratio are not maturity indicators. To obtain the
necessary data, extensive trials were made involving
proportional dividers, vernier calipers and clear plastic rulers, graduated to 0.5 mm or 1.0 mm.[**] These
trials showed that the rulers were best in regard to
repeatability, comparability, ease of handling, time
required for training, and possible damage to the
radiographs. By calculating correlation coefficients
between these ratios and chronological age, across all
ages, it was shown that ratios based on the original
measurements would be more useful than those based on
logs of these measurements.

Throughout the study, several assessors tested
possible indicators and used those considered useful
to grade radiographs. During these procedures, dis-
cussions between assessors were frequent and both
repeatability and comparability were tested systematically. As a result of these tests, the methodology of
assessment was standardized and the descriptions of the
indicators clarified. It is realized that often there
will be less opportunity for discussion when others
apply the present method.

Although each assessor can measure his repeatability, by rating groups of radiographs more than once,
it is more difficult to obtain the cooperation of colleagues, that is needed to monitor comparability.
Because of this problem, considerable attention has been

[*] Ellipse Master No. 2078, Arthur Brown and Bro., Inc.
     2 West 46th Street, New York, N.Y. 10036.

[**] Available from C-THRU Ruler Company, 6 Britton Drive,
     Bloomfield, Conn., 06002 (No. B-55).

given to providing clear brief written descriptions of
indicators, employing a standardized anatomical
terminology. These descriptions have been supplemented
by photographs and drawings of the alternative appearances to which the same grade is assigned. Furthermore,
copies of 20 radiographs, covering the whole range of
maturity levels, have been prepared for training
purposes.*

The raw data were recorded cross-sectionally,
without reference to earlier or later serial radiographs, so that the final system would be applicable
when only one radiograph of a child was available.
In this recording, there was no bias from knowledge of
what had been observed in other radiographs of the same
child. However, as will be described, the cross-
sectional data were analyzed serially to determine the
validity of possible maturity indicators (See Step 4, iv;
pp. 77-79).

Step 4. Because many possible indicators had to
be tested, screening procedures were adopted to allow
rapid identification of "indicators" that were clearly
not useful. For the first screening, use was made of
serial radiographs of 8 boys (primary test group) who
attended for each scheduled examination during the age
range for which the indicator was considered potentially
useful. These radiographs were graded twice by two
assessors working independently. At the end of this
procedure, many "indicators" were rejected. This step
greatly simplified the method of assessment.

The definitions of some of the indicators, that
were retained, were rewritten to remove ambiguity or
because unexpected variations in form had been observed
in the radiographs. In grading some curvatures, it was
found necessary to alter the length of each constructed
curve or to reduce the number of curves used. Due to

* Sets of these copies, together with the grades
  assigned to each indicator and the distances used
  to derive ratios, are available from the first author.

these changes in the descriptions of the grades, the radiographs in the primary test group were rated again.

Each indicator had to satisfy five criteria to be regarded as useful. Because the primary test group was small, only definite failure to meet a criterion was regarded as a basis for omitting further testing. When this occurred, an indicator was not tested further unless the definition of grades was modified. If such changes were made, the modified indicator was retested.

The criteria applied to test data from the primary test group concerned:

(i) Discrimination. This is the ability of an indicator to assist in distinguishing between children

TABLE XII

Constructed Curves Used to Grade Indicators

Indicators	Length of Curve (mm)	Pole	Length of Ellipse (mm)	Degrees of Ellipse	Designation
FEM-H (1)	6	Major	22	50	I
FEM-H (2)	8	Minor	15	50	II
FEM-H (3)	8	Minor	22	20	III
TIB-L (1,2)	7	Major	22	50	IV
TIB-J (1,2)	7	Major	15	50	V
TIB-K (1,2)	7	Major	22	30	VI

The figures in brackets refer to the grades of the indicators.

of the same chronological age. If an "indicator,"
e.g., the indentation in the articular surface of the
femoral epiphysis, occurs in all boys aged 10 years, it
cannot assist the assessment of skeletal maturity at
this chronological age. The indicator may, however,
assist discrimination at other ages. The ability of
indicators to discriminate was judged from the prevalence of different grades in groups of test radiographs
at various chronological ages. Test data for indicators
based on ratios were examined to determine whether they
were sufficiently variable, within chronological age

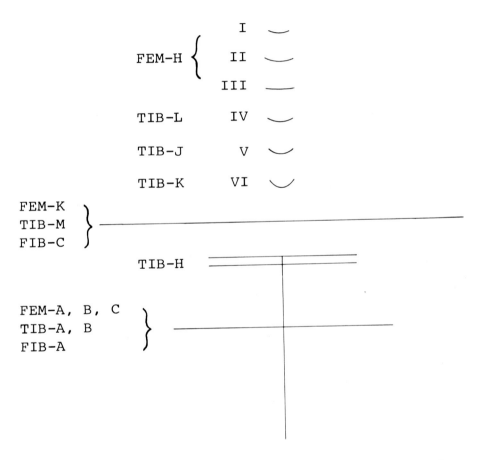

Figure 14. Standard curves, straight lines and a 2 mm
gap for use in grading indicators. These are provided
on clear plastic in the back of the book. Extra copies
may be obtained from Dr. Alex Roche.

groups, to assist discrimination. It is stressed that
the present description of the way in which this and
other criteria were applied relates to data from the
primary test group of 8 boys.

(ii) <u>Universality</u>. By definition, each grade of
every indicator must occur during the maturation of an
individual. In indicators that have multiple grades,
the incidence of intermediate grades need not reach
100 percent at any age because children differ in their
rates of maturation. Thus, in a five grade indicator,
some 10 year old boys may be at grade 2 and others at
grade 3 and there may be no earlier or later age when
either grade 2 or grade 3 is universal. However, both
the least mature and the most mature grades must be
universal at some ages. This might be clarified by
using **FEM-D** as an example. Briefly, the three grades
of the shape of the femoral epiphysis are:

Grade 1 -- elliptical
Grade 2 -- ovoid
Grade 3 -- indented.

The intermediate grade (grade 2) was not universal
at any age (Table **XIII**) although review of serial radiographs showed that the sequence in all children was
grade 1 $\longrightarrow$ grade 2 $\longrightarrow$ grade 3.

Serial radiographs extending to 24 years were
graded when universality had not been established by
18 years to test the universality of grades that
appear late.

As far as possible, the criterion of universality
was applied also to indicators based on ratios by
examining the data to see if the values became approximately constant at older ages. The test data for these
indicators were examined to determine whether the ratios
were the same, or almost the same, in all the primary
test group boys just prior to epiphyseo-diaphyseal
fusion. Some of the measurements required for indicators based on ratios could not be made at later ages
because not all limits of the epiphyses and the
metaphyses could be recognized.

(iii) <u>Reliability.</u> The aspects of reliability used as criteria were comparability and repeatability. The radiographs in the primary test group were assessed twice by two observers working independently. The data were pooled across age within three age ranges (one month through 4 years; 4.5 through 10 years and 11 through 18 years). Comparability was determined from interobserver differences and repeatability was judged from intraobserver differences. Arbitrarily, the indicators were considered reliable if the incidence of both interobserver and intraobserver differences in the grades assigned was less than 8 percent. The reliability of indicators based on ratios was considered acceptable if the mean absolute interobserver and intraobserver differences for the measurements used to derive these ratios were each less than 0.5 mm.

TABLE XIII

The Percentage Prevalence
of Grades of FEM-D
in Boys

Age in months	Grades		
	1	2	3
1	96	4	0
3	76	23	1
6	21	77	2
9	1	78	21
12	0	49	51
18	0	12	88
24	0	0	100

(iv) <u>Validity.</u> An indicator being tested may discriminate, become universal, and be reliable but may not indicate maturity. In the present context, validity refers to the quality by which a radiographic appearance indicates skeletal maturity. If this quality is absent, the indicator lacks validity.

It has been claimed that the validity of skeletal age assessments can be shown by an increase in the accuracy of predictions of age at epiphyseo-diaphyseal fusion as predictions are made at more advanced skeletal ages (Flory, 1938). This test has not been applied. When one considers the size of the errors involved in the estimation of the skeletal age of the knee, there is no real possibility that one single indicator could predict the timing of a later indicator across a reasonable time interval.

An alternative method is to review data from serial radiographs. A priori, the bones of a child must become more mature with increasing chronological age although indicators of this increased maturity may not be visible radiographically. Therefore, as pointed out by Takahashi (1956), the prevalence of grades of valid maturity indicators must change systematically with age until the most mature grade is universal. Corresponding progressive alterations must occur in the ratios used as indicators. Prevalence data for grades of qualitative indicators and changes in mean ratios from a group of children studied serially can provide a general guide to validity but (because children miss visits) a better measure is obtained by reviewing serial data for individuals.

In the present study, the basic readings for each indicator were made "cross-sectionally," i.e., without reference to earlier or later radiographs of the child. However, the radiographs were serial and the data for individuals were subsequently reviewed across age. "Reversals" were sought in these serially organized data; i.e., changes in indicators with increasing age that were in the reverse direction to those expected from the group trends. These changes involved the

grades assigned. In the indicators based on ratios,
a similar principal was adopted after the continua of
values for these ratios had been divided to categories
(Table XIV).

The incidence of reversals was considered in two
ways: first, as the percentage of children in whom they
were observed, and secondly, as the percentage of
observed/possible reversals. The number of possible
reversals for the group = $\sum$ (N-1) where N = number of
radiographs for each child. The second of these percentages is the more important because the first is a
function of the number of radiographs per child.
Indicator grades may be skipped in serial data for an
individual. This may not be due to a lack of validity
but to a schedule in which the intervals between radiographs were too long.

TABLE XIV

Limits of Categories Assigned to Grades Based on Ratios

Indicators	Categories				
	1	2	3	4	5
FEM-A	<0.50	0.51-0.60	0.61-0.70	0.71-0.80	>0.80
FEM-B	<2.00	2.01-2.25	2.26-2.50	2.51-2.75	>2.75
FEM-C	<1.00	1.01-1.10	1.11-1.20	1.21-1.30	>1.30
TIB-A	<0.60	0.61-0.70	0.71-0.80	0.81-0.90	>0.90
TIB-B	<2.50	2.51-2.70	2.71-2.90	2.91-3.10	>3.10
FIB-A	<0.30	0.31-0.50	0.51-0.70	0.71-0.90	>0.90

"Maturity indicators" with a high incidence of possible reversals (> 15%) were omitted because, in fact, they did not indicate maturity even if they met all the other criteria considered in Step 4.

The practice adopted is similar to that of Hughes and Tanner (1970) who wrote: "A high incidence of reversals would have been undesirable as this would have indicated that the stages were too finely spaced and the error in assigning a rating would be high. It was equally undesirable to have no reversals at all as this would have indicated that the stages were too coarse and therefore of less than optimal use for detecting the smaller changes in skeletal maturity."

When a clinician assesses a single radiograph using the present RWT method or the atlas method (Greulich and Pyle, 1959; Pyle and Hoerr, 1969), the fact that maturity indicators occasionally show reversals will be of no concern. However, when serial radiographs of an individual are being assessed, reversals can cause concern. Generally the reversals are due to slight variations in film density or radiographic positioning. If the clinician is convinced that the reversal is artifactual, he should assign to the latter radiograph the more mature grade, or ratio, that was assigned to the earlier radiograph. It is stressed that these reversals occur in individual indicators and that they were uncommon in those finally chosen. Reversals did not occur in the serial RWT skeletal ages for the knee joint.

(v) Completeness. This criterion is the extent to which each indicator could be recorded in the primary test sample. Application of this criterion did not lead to the exclusion of any indicator but it did restrict the age ranges during which some indicators should be recorded. For example, transverse trabeculae in the femoral epiphysis (FEM-G) can be seen in few radiographs of boys aged more than 14 years although they are universally present before this. The reason is that the cortical bone becomes so radio-opaque that they are obscured.

The above criteria were considered separately for each indicator. The question of redundancy was not investigated in the selection of useful indicators. However, in the mathematical estimation procedures that were applied later, each indicator was weighted depending upon the information it provided (Chapter V).

Because many possible indicators had to be tested, screening procedures were adopted to allow rapid identification of "indicators" that were clearly not useful. For the first screening, use was made of serial radiographs of 8 boys (<u>primary test group</u>) who attended for each scheduled examination during the age range for which the indicator was considered potentially useful. These radiographs were graded twice by two assessors working independently. At the end of this procedure, many "indicators" were rejected as useless. The definitions of other indicators were rewritten to remove ambiguity or because unexpected variations had been observed in the radiographs. In grading some curvatures, it was necessary to alter the length of each constructed curve or to reduce the number of curves used. These changes in descriptions and grades necessitated regrading the primary test group.

Because the primary test group was small, only definite failure to meet a criterion was regarded as a basis for omitting further testing. When this occurred, an indicator was not tested further unless the definition of grades was modified. After such changes were made, the modified indicator was retested.

If the findings from the primary test group were equivocal or satisfactory, the indicator was retained for the next phase of testing. As stated earlier, when one criterion or more were definitely not met in the test radiographs, it was considered that the indicator was not useful and it was not tested further. Before this exclusion, the primary test data were considered carefully to determine the factors responsible for the apparent lack of usefulness. On many occasions, this led to reassessments and the adoption of procedures designed to exclude the effects of such factors as:

(a) unreliability of ratings by a particular assessor. In such cases, the assessor received further instruction and training.

(b) unreliability due to the difficulty of distinguishing between particular grades. Usually the number of grades was decreased; sometimes grades were redefined.

(c) variations in radiographic positioning. With many indicators, it was found necessary to use only knee radiographs. Others were substituted only after they had passed the test procedures described earlier (p.65).

(d) age-associated problems. The data for some indicators showed that the criteria were met at some ages but not others. When such difficulties were encountered during testing, in the indicators finally chosen, they were due to the factors considered under (b) and (c).

Step 5.   Some indicators with two grades were combined, resulting in a smaller number of indicators with multiple grades. For example, three theoretical preliminary indicators may have been:

Indicator 1. The epiphysis is ossified.

      Grade 1 -- absent
      Grade 2 -- present

Indicator 2. The ossified part of the epiphysis
      is circular with a diameter of about 1 mm.

      Grade 1 -- absent
      Grade 2 -- present

Indicator 3. The ossified epiphyseal area is
      elliptical.

      Grade 1 -- absent
      Grade 2 -- present

These three dichotomous indicators would have been
combined to a single indicator with three grades:

    Grade 1 -- the epiphysis is not ossified
    Grade 2 -- the ossified part of the epiphysis
               is circular with a diameter of
               about 1 mm
    Grade 3 -- the ossified part of the epiphysis
               is elliptical.

Such combinations removed much redundant information
and made recording simpler. As experience was gained,
some preliminary dichotomous indicators were combined
to indicators with multiple grades prior to testing.

    Step 6. The indicators not eliminated previously
were recorded in a secondary test group of radiographs
of 20 boys, at each age, who had not been included in
the primary test group. These radiographs were graded
twice by two assessors working independently. In general, these were the same assessors who had tested
the indicator earlier; if not, they received appropriate training.

    The data from the secondary test group were
analyzed for reliability (comparability and repeatability) and completeness. Validity, discrimination
and universality were tested later, using data from
the whole sample. Some indicators that had appeared
of doubtful usefulness after the primary testing were
excluded because they failed to meet the necessary
criteria when they were applied to the secondary test
group. The findings from the secondary test group led
to further modifications in the descriptions of useful
indicators and to changes in the age ranges during
which they appeared to be useful.

    As a result of these testing procedures, only
about 15 percent of the "maturity indicators" described
in the literature were retained. There remained 34
useful indicators for the femur, tibia and fibula;
none of these were applicable throughout the whole
range of maturity levels. It is very important that

TABLE XV

Percentage Incidence of Reversals (Validity)

FEMUR

FEM	BOYS	GIRLS
A	1.0	0.9
B	1.5	0.1
C	2.4	4.6
D	1.3	2.1
E	7.5	0.0
F	9.6	10.2
G	13.8	11.2
H	10.0	12.8
J	3.7	6.5
K	4.6	6.2
L	7.3	2.1
M	4.6	5.6

In this table, and in Tables XVI and XVII, the prevalence of reversals was calculated for the age range from when the least mature grade was present in 75 percent of the children to when the most mature grade was present in 75 percent of the children except for those based on ratios (FEM-A, -B, -C, TIB-A, -B, and FIB-A). In the latter, the whole appropriate age range was used before they were changed to graded categories.

judgments of skeletal maturity be based only on indicators shown to be satisfactory. This saves time and can
provide a more accurate estimate.

Step 7. All suitable radiographs of boys were
graded for each apparently useful indicator except
that the secondary test group (20 boys) was not graded
again. When more than one radiograph of the knee
area of a boy was available at a particular age, only
one was assessed.

Step 8. The data from the whole group were
analyzed in relation to universality, validity and
completeness. To determine validity, the incidence of
reversals (as a percentage of those possible) was calculated for each indicator for the age range from when
the least mature grade was present in 75 percent of
the children to when the most mature grade was present
in 75 percent of the children. This range was chosen
to represent more accurately the validity of each
indicator by excluding age ranges during which it was
very commonly absent or very commonly present. Among
the finally chosen indicators, the median incidence of
reversals was 4.4 percent (Tables XV-XVII).

A few indicators were excluded after this step,
although they had been graded in all radiographs.
This occurred whenever it was shown that they were not
useful although they had met all the criteria applied
to the data from the primary and secondary test groups.

Step 9. The data relating to the grades of the
indicators (prevalence across age) for the whole sample
of boys were graphed on probability paper. These
graphs were used for the following purposes:

(a) to estimate the approximate age at which the
prevalence of each indicator grade reached 50 percent.
When the prevalence did not reach this level in the
recorded data the age range of the observations was
extended or, when appropriate, adjoining grades were
combined and the description of the indicators modified.
Some intermediate grades were retained even if they did

TABLE XVI

Percentage Incidence of Reversals (Validity)

TIBIA

TIB	BOYS	GIRLS
A	0.4	0.5
B	8.4	5.8
C	5.2	2.3
D	6.1	5.8
E	7.6	9.1
F	12.2	13.1
G	2.3	5.5
H	3.7	3.7
J	0.6	4.4
K	6.0	6.0
L	13.3	13.9
M	7.5	7.6
N	2.2	1.5
P	1.1	0.4
Q	2.6	2.0
R	2.3	3.7

not reach a 50 percent prevalence at any age. This was
done when there were useful grades before and after the
intermediate grade and its retention increased the
separation between the ages at which the earlier and
later grades reached 50 percent prevalence levels.

This can be illustrated with data relating to
indicator FEM-L (Table XVIII). This indicator refers
to fusion in the lateral part of the epiphyseo-diaphyseal
junction. Grade 1 reaches the 50 percent prevalence
level between 16 and 17 years, grade 2 does not reach
the 50 percent level at any age and grade 3 reaches
this level between 17 and 18 years. Because grades 1
and 3 reach the 50 percent levels at different ages
they supply independent information. However, if
grades 2 and 3 were combined, this new grade (2 + 3)
would have percentage prevalences that were the recip-
rocals of those for grade 1. This compound grade would
reach the 50 percent level at the same age as grade 1

TABLE XVII

Percentage Incidence of Reversals (Validity)

FIBULA

FIB	BOYS	GIRLS
A	1.4	0.9
B	6.3	3.8
C	1.3	2.0
D	11.4	7.8
E	3.2	2.7
F	2.0	4.0

and its slope would be the same as that for grade 1 except that the sign would be different. This compound grade (2 + 3) would not provide independent information.

(b) to judge the rate of change across age in the prevalence of each indicator grade. Indicator grades with more rapid changes in prevalence, especially near the age when the grade is present in 50 percent of the sample, provide more precise estimates of skeletal maturity.

(c) to appraise the regularity of changes in prevalence across age. When these were irregular, the cause was sought. If they were associated with variations in the types of radiographs used, some data were excluded. If they were due to the lack of reliability

TABLE XVIII

Percentage Incidence of Grades
of FEM-L in Boys

Age	Final grades			Grades 2+3
(years)	1	2	3	combined
11	100	0	0	0
12	96	4	0	4
13	95	5	0	5
14	91	9	0	9
15	73	26	1	27
16	58	33	9	42
17	19	41	40	81
18	9	19	72	91

of a particular assessor, further training was provided
and the radiographs were regraded. In other instances,
the indicator was redefined and rated again.

(d) to determine the age ranges over which the
indicators discriminate. This was defined arbitrarily
as the range within which the prevalence of the most
common grade was less than 98 percent.

Step 10. Chapter V describes the statistical
basis for the scoring procedures by which data from
each indicator are used to measure skeletal maturity.
In summary, the first step was to change the continuous
ratios into five categories for each indicator. The
limits of these categories are given in Table XIV.

This categorization introduces very little loss of
information and greatly reduces measurement error.
After this transformation, all the data were in the
form of ordered categories that could be combined into
a single continuous index through the use of latent
trait analysis (Birnbaum, 1968; Samejima, 1969, 1972).

This index, which exists at all relevant ages,
was scaled to years. The resulting model is con-
strained across ages, so that, in the group from whom
the scale is derived, the mean and the variance of
skeletal age is the mean and the variance of chronological age. The extent to which individuals in a
particular age group differ in skeletal age is an
aspect of particular interest.

The statistical method that was applied allows
the separation of the within age variance into two
components. One is attributable to real variations in
maturity level. The second is attributable to error
which is inherent in any scheme. This is the only
statistical method yet developed which estimates this
second error component in data of the present type.

The parameters of the model for each indicator
grade used in the construction of the new scale are
the chronological age at which it is present in

50 percent of the boys and the rate of change in prevalence with age; these data are obtained from logit
analyses.

The skeletal age estimation procedure (Appendix II)
requires, as input data, the grade of each indicator,
and the sex of the child. The output from the program
is the estimated skeletal age in years, with the
standard error of this estimate. The program does not
require that each indicator be graded. However, if
some indicators appropriate for the age of the child
are omitted, the skeletal age estimate will be less
precise; this will be reflected in a larger standard
error of the estimate. Indicator grades that are not
yet present must be so scored; those that are not
scored because the child is too young (immature) or too
old (mature) most be recorded differently. The ability
of individual indicators to provide information about
skeletal maturity is shown, at each maturity level, by
the inverse of their error at that maturity level.
Although some are generally more informative than others,
all the indicators that met the set criteria were
retained.

Extension of the Method to Girls

After Steps 1 through 9 had been completed for
the boys, the method was applied to girls. It was
decided to omit, without further testing, the indicators that were not useful in boys. Each indicator that
had been shown to be useful in boys was tested, using
a primary test group of serial radiographs of 8 girls
and a secondary test group of serial radiographs of
20 other girls.

This testing had several purposes. Some of those
assessing the radiographs of girls had no prior experience with certain indicators; the testing process
provided this. Analyses of data from both the primary
and secondary test groups showed that each indicator
finally chosen for the girls met every criterion that
had been applied to the indicators when they had been

tested in the boys. The adductor tubercle was marginally useful in the boys. In the boys, it did meet
all the criteria but reversals were relatively common
and the change in prevalence with age was very slow.
Because it did not become universal in the girls, it
was not included among the indicators that were finally
chosen for either sex.

It was assumed that each indicator should be
graded during younger age ranges in the girls than the
boys because, as is well known, skeletal maturation
typically proceeds more rapidly in girls than in boys.
The testing process confirmed this and provided a useful
guide to the extent of this difference. When the
recorded data for the indicators in the whole sample of
girls were transferred to probability graph paper, it
was found necessary to extend some of the age ranges
during which the data had been recorded. For example,
if the most mature grade of an indicator became universal in boys at 11 years, this indicator would not have
been recorded in girls after 9 years. However, when
the data were reviewed, it was noted often that the
indicator had not become universal and it was necessary
to rate the girls at additional ages (9.5, 10.0,....
years) until the indicator did become universal.

In summary, the testing procedures in the girls
provided training and they helped define the age range
for recording each indicator. This testing showed that
all the indicators for boys were useful for girls
except the adductor tubercle, which, as noted earlier,
did not become universal in girls at any age.

CHAPTER IV

THE FINAL MATURITY INDICATORS

All illustrations are from anteroposterior radio-graphs of left knees. Consequently, the lateral margin is on the left hand side of each illustration. A star ★ at the top of the page describing an indicator shows that the plastic sheet (enclosed in the back of this book or obtainable from Dr. Alex Roche) should be used for rating a radiograph.

FEMORAL INDICATORS

These indicators met all the criteria that were
applied. It is stressed that considerable variation
was found and that few, if any, of the radiographic
shadows conformed exactly to the geometric terms used
to define some of the indicators. Consequently, drawings and photographic reproductions have been included
to assist an appreciation of the range of shapes to
which the same grade was assigned. Radiographs in
which the knee is rotated should not be assessed by the
present method. In the descriptions of indicators, the
term "midline" refers to a bone and not necessarily
the midline of the knee.

The description of each indicator includes the age
ranges during which it is useful in boys and girls.
As would be expected, these ranges tend to be later in
the boys. These useful age ranges have been defined
generously. At earlier or later ages the indicators
are not likely to be useful in normal children. In
clinical circumstances, however, it could be necessary
to assign indicator grades outside the age ranges given.
A list of femoral indicators, with the appropriate age
ranges for normal children, is given in Table XIX.

TABLE   XIX

Summary of Indicators for Distal End of Femur

Indicator	Description	Grades	Age range
FEM-A	Ratio EW/MW	5	Boys:1 mo.-6.5 yr. Girls:1 mo.-5.5 yr.
FEM-B	Ratio EW/EH	5	Boys: 1-6 years Girls:9 mo.-5.5 yr.
FEM-C	Ratio WLC/HLC	5	Boys: 1-5.5 yr. Girls:9 mo.-3.5 yr.
FEM-D	Epiphyseal shape	3	Boys: 1 mo.-2 yr. Girls: 1 mo.-2 yr.
FEM-E	Terminal plate	2	Boys:1 mo.-2.5 yr. Girls:1 mo.- 2 yr.
FEM-F	Radio-opaque lateral margin of medial condyle	2	Boys:5.5-18 years Girls:3-13 years
FEM-G	Transverse trabeculae	2	Boys:5.5-14 years Girls: 4-15 years
FEM-H	Lateral articular margin	3	Boys: 1-11 years Girls:9 mo.-11 yr.
FEM-J	Shape of proximo-lateral corner of epiphysis	2	Boys: 5-17 years Girls:4.5-11 years
FEM-K	Lateral capping	3	Boys: 8-17 years Girls:7.5-16 years
FEM-L	Lateral fusion	3	Boys: 11-18 years Girls:11-18 years
FEM-M	Medial fusion	3	Boys: 11-18 years Girls: 9-18 years

EW = epiphyseal width; MW = metaphyseal width;
EH = epiphyseal height; WLC = width of lateral condyle,
and HLC = height of lateral condyle.

FEM-A ★

Ratio $\dfrac{\text{epiphyseal width}}{\text{metaphyseal width}}$

Boys: 1 month to 6.5 years
Girls: 1 month to 5.5 years

The measurements used in each ratio (FEM-A, FEM-B, and FEM-C) are made using a clear plastic rule graduated to 0.5 mm. They are recorded to the nearest 0.5 mm. The widths of both the epiphysis and the metaphysis are measured as maximum widths at right angles to the long axis of the femoral diaphysis (Fig. 15). Irregularities of the epiphyseal margin are included but areas of disseminated calcification are excluded.

This ratio should not be recorded in children with rickets. Despite this limitation, it has been retained because it is so informative at younger ages. FEM-A can be assessed only when an ossified epiphysis is present but fusion has not occurred.

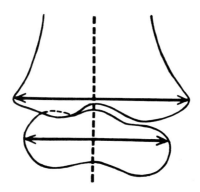

Figure 15. The planes in which epiphyseal and metaphyseal widths of the femur are measured.

FEM-D

Epiphyseal shape: 3 grades

                              Boys: 1 month to 2 years
                              Girls: 1 month to 2 years

        Grade 1 -- elliptical

        Grade 2 -- ovoid

        Grade 3 -- indentation present

    Careful inspection is necessary when this indica-
tor is being graded because parts of the epiphysis may
be only slightly radio-opaque.

    In Grade 1 the epiphyseal outline is elliptical
with its long axis transverse (Figs. 18-19). Rarely, if
ever, does the outline exactly match the geometric
definition of elliptical. The range of shapes to which
this grade is assigned is illustrated in Figure 18.
Clearly, size is not a factor in rating. Minor irregularities in the shape of the margin are disregarded.

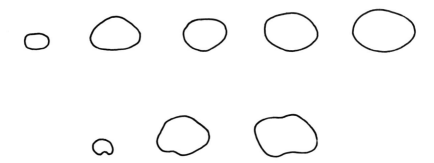

Figure 18. Shapes to which Grade 1 of FEM-D is assigned.

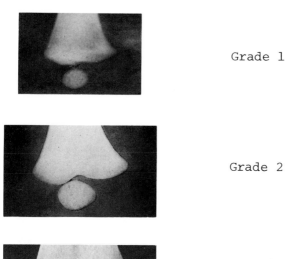

Grade 1

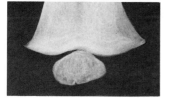

Grade 2

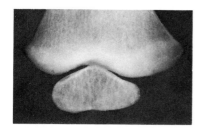

Grade 2

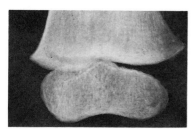

Grade 3
Slight

Grade 3
Marked

Figure 19.   Examples of FEM-D.

Grade 2 is assigned when the epiphyseal outline is ovoid, with the lateral end blunter than the medial (Figs.19 and 20). Some epiphyseal outlines are ovoid except that they are flattened on their distal or articular margins (Fig. 20). When this appearance is present, Grade 2 is assigned.

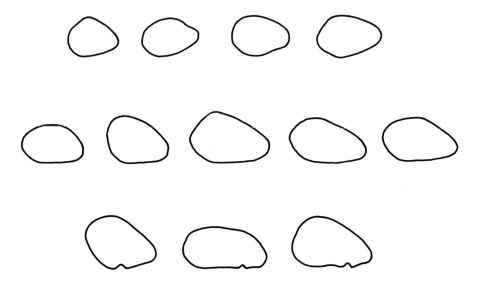

Figure 20.   Shapes to which Grade 2 of FEM-D is assigned.

In Grade 3, the distal (articular) margin of the
epiphysis is indented near the midline (Figs. 19 and 21).
An indentation is considered present if part of this
margin, near the midline, is proximal to a tangent to
the lateral and medial parts of the margin and, therefore, concave distally. Examples of slight, moderate
and marked indentations are shown in Figure 21.
In unusual radiographs, there are deep narrow notches
in the articular margin (Fig. 20). These are assigned
Grade 2 because these clefts occur in epiphyses that
have generally irregular margins and a review of serial
radiographs showed that indentations form later independently of these clefts.

The various grades of FEM-D are assigned independently of whether the epiphyseal outline is regular or
irregular as long as the irregularity is not more marked
than indicated in Figures 18-21. If it is more irregular, the epiphysis cannot be graded but this is very
unusual. There may be a radio-opaque line near the
margin of this epiphysis (Sontag, 1938) but this is not
used in grading.

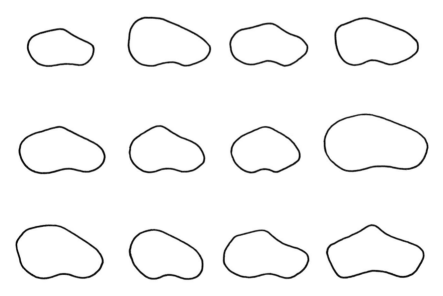

Figure 21.   Shapes to which Grade 3 of FEM-D are
assigned.

FEM-E

Terminal plate: 2 grades

                                    Boys: 1 month to 2.5 years
                                    Girls: 1 month to 2 years

            Grade 1 -- absent

            Grade 2 -- present

      The terminal plate causes a thin radio-opaque line
that remains on the metaphyseal margin of the epiphyseal
shadow until fusion.

      Grade 1 is recorded when this line is completely
absent or it occupies less than one quarter of the
margin.

      Grade 2 is recorded when a terminal plate is
related to one quarter or more of the metaphyseal margin of the epiphysis. Usually the terminal plate is
noted first medial to the midline of the epiphysis.
It may appear continuous with the shadow caused by well
defined cortical bone on the lateral or the medial non-
articular margins of the epiphysis. Occasionally the
radio-opaque line due to the terminal plate is interrupted (Fig. 22). In a few younger children, superimposed shadows, especially in the lateral part of the
epiphysis, make it difficult to decide whether a terminal plate is present and, in extreme cases, it may be
impossible to assess this indicator.

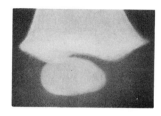

Grade 1

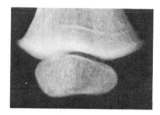

Grade 2
Interrupted

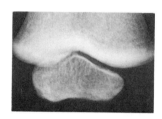

Grade 2
Incomplete

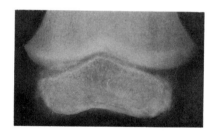

Grade 2
Complete

Figure 22.   Examples of FEM-E.

FEM-F

Radio-opaque lateral margin of medial condyle: 2 grades

Boys: 5.5 to 18 years
Girls: 3 to 13 years

Grade 1 -- absent

Grade 2 -- present

The position of this radio-opaque line is shown in Figure 23.

Grade 2 is recorded when the radio-opaque line extends over at least half the distance between the articular and metaphyseal margins. This line is seen first in the central part of the epiphysis between

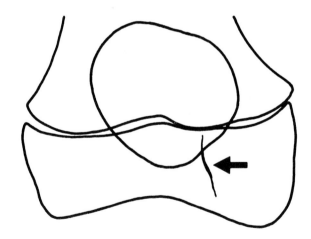

Figure 23. The position of the radio-opaque line due to the lateral margin of the medial condyle.

these two margins.   Later it usually extends to both the
articular and metaphyseal margins.   It is approximately
vertical and can be distinguished from vertical trabeculae because it is wider (Fig. 24).   This indicator
can be assessed only after there is an indentation in
the articular margin of the epiphysis (FEM-D; Grade 3).

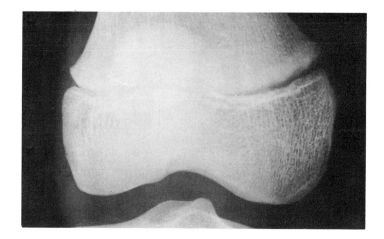

Grade 1

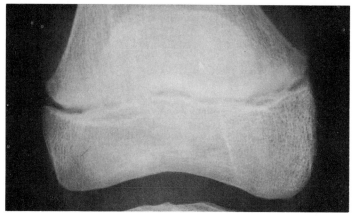

Grade 2

Figure 24.   Examples of FEM-F.

FEM-G

Transverse trabeculae: 2 grades

Boys: 5.5 to 14 years
Girls: 4 to 15 years

Grade 1 -- absent

Grade 2 -- present

The position of these transverse trabeculae is
shown in Figure 25.

This trabecular pattern is approximately transverse,
radiating medially from near the midline of the epiphysis (Fig. 25). Grade 2 is assigned only when the transverse trabeculae extend as far as the radio-opaque line
caused by the lateral margin of the medial condyle
(FEM-F), or as far as the area where this line occurs.

Commonly, this indicator cannot be assessed after
13 years because the cortical and cancellous bone cause
dense shadows that obscure the trabeculae.

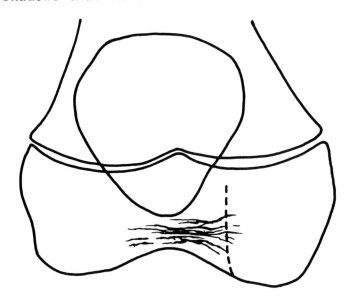

Figure 25.   The position of the transverse trabeculae.

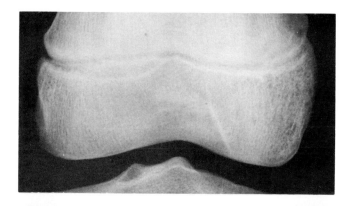

Grade 1

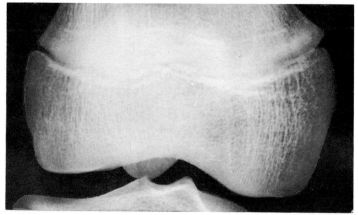

Grade 1
Incomplete

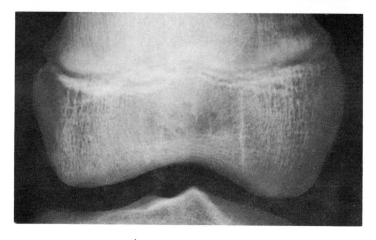

Grade 2

Figure 26.   Examples of FEM-G.

General Notes Regarding Curve Fitting

Several indicators for the femur and tibia relate
to the curvature of part of the margin of the ossified
part of an epiphysis. Any grading scheme artificially
divides the continuum of the curvatures that exists in
a series of radiographs. To grade curvatures as objectively as possible, geometric curves, drawn on transparent plastic, are matched with the part of the
epiphyseal margin to be graded. The plastic sheet is
moved across the radiograph to fit a curve to the part
of the margin being graded. Minor irregularities of
the margin, including slight disseminated calcification,
are disregarded; the general form is graded.

The most accurate method is to place the ends of
each curve on the margin with the midpoint of the curve
opposite the area being assessed. The next step is to
appraise the congruence of the margin and the central
part of the curve. A slightly different procedure is
used when curves are fitted to the tibial tubercles
(TIB-J and TIB-K). Each curve is the minor or major
pole of an ellipse (Figure 27).

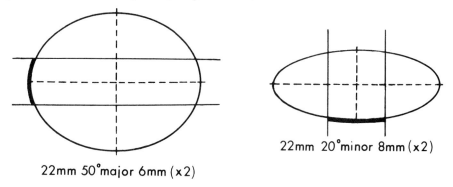

22mm 50°major 6mm (x2)   22mm 20°minor 8mm (x2)

Figure 27. The thick parts of these ellipses show
curves derived from minor and major poles.

FEM-H ★

Curvature of lateral part of articular surface: 3 grades

                              Boys: 1 to 11 years
                              Girls: 9 months to 11 years

    Grade 1 -- as curved or more curved than Standard
Curve I (6 mm long; major pole; 22 mm; 50°)

    Grade 2 -- similar in curvature to Standard Curve II
(8 mm long; minor pole; 15 mm; 50°)

    Grade 3 -- as curved or flatter than Standard
Curve III (8 mm long; minor pole; 22 mm; 20°)

    If the curvature is judged to be midway between
two grades, the more mature grade is assigned. The
part of the margin to which the curves are fitted is
shown in Figure 28. It is important that the curve be
placed so that its midpoint is opposite the midpoint of
the lateral part of the articular surface. At younger
ages but not later, the midpoint of this surface is
also its most distal point (Fig. 28).

    In grading FEM-H, the least mature grade is
assigned to the most sharply curved margin. This
indicator cannot be graded until an indentation is
present (FEM-D; Grade 3). It cannot be assessed satisfactorily in lower leg radiographs.

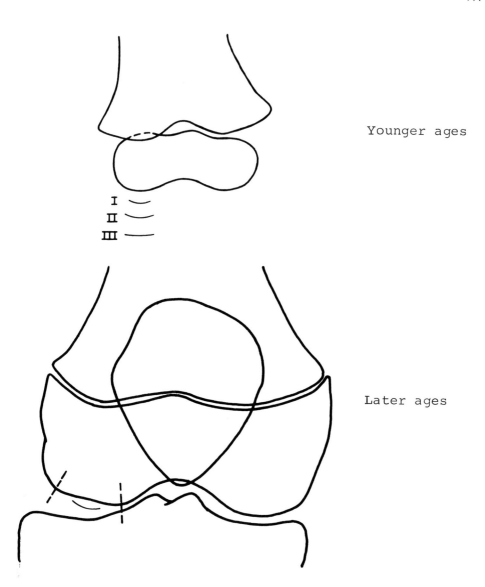

I
II
III

Younger ages

Later ages

Figure 28. The way in which curves are fitted to Grade FEM-H at earlier and later ages.

FEM-K ★

Lateral capping: 3 grades

                              Boys: 8 to 17 years
                              Girls: 7.5 to 16 years

        Grade 1 -- absent

        Grade 2 -- incomplete

        Grade 3 -- complete

    "Capping" refers to the way in which the epiphysis
overlaps the metaphysis as maturation proceeds. This
occurs at the junction between the lateral and distal
margins of the metaphysis. Commonly, this junction is
bevelled; less often it is convex.

    The grading of this indicator is most reliable
when it is based on the following procedure. A straight
line on transparent plastic is placed as a tangent to
the two parts of the end of the metaphysis (medial and
lateral to the midline) that are convex distally
(Fig. 30). The plastic is moved across the radiograph,
keeping the line parallel to this tangent to the end of
the metaphysis, until the line passes through the distal end of the bevelled area (site of capping) on the
metaphysis.

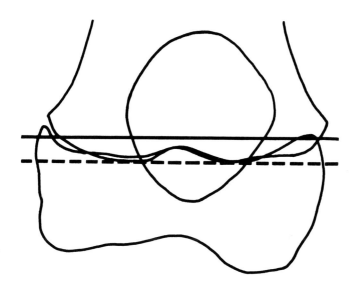

Figure 30. To grade FEM-K, a tangent (-----) placed
across the end of the metaphysis is moved proximally,
in the same plane, to the position of the solid
line (_____).

Grade 2 is assigned if the epiphysis extends proximal to this line and <u>in relation to part of the bevelled area</u>.

Grade 3 is assigned if the epiphysis extends proximal to this line and <u>in relation to all the bevelled area</u> (Fig. 31).

Occasionally, there are two radio-opaque lines on or near the lateral margin of the metaphysis just proximal to the bevelled area. These are not used in grading. If fusion is complete at the lateral end of the epiphyseo-metaphyseal junction (**FEM-L, Grade 3**) this indicator is not assessed.

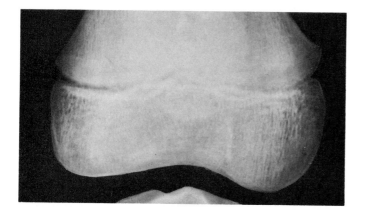

Grade 1

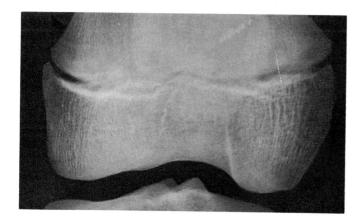

Grade 2

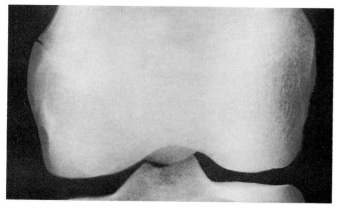

Grade 3

Figure 31.   Examples of FEM-K.

FEM-L

Lateral epiphyseo-metaphyseal fusion: 3 grades

                                        Boys: 11 to 18 years
                                        Girls: 11 to 18 years

        Grade 1 -- absent

        Grade 2 -- incomplete

        Grade 3 -- complete

    The lateral part of the epiphyseo-metaphyseal
junction extends from the lateral margins of the
epiphysis and metaphysis to the most distal point on
the lateral half of the metaphyseal margin. The part
of the junction near the midline is not graded because
it is difficult to interpret due to overlapping shadows including those due to the patella.

Grade 1 is assigned when there is a relatively radiolucent strip, or several discontinuous strips that overlap and collectively extend for the whole length of the lateral part of the junction (Fig. 32). If there are complete terminal plates on both the metaphysis and epiphysis, fusion is not present.

Grade 2 is recorded when definite bony fusion is seen across part but not all of the lateral portion of the junction. The best evidence of fusion is absence of a radiolucent epiphyseal zone.

Grade 3 is assigned when fusion is complete in the lateral part of the junction, without any notch at the lateral end. The radio-opaque line of fusion may be visible.

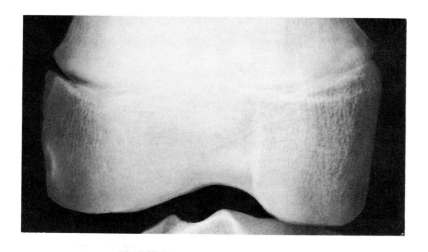

Figure 32.   FEM-L -- Grade 1.

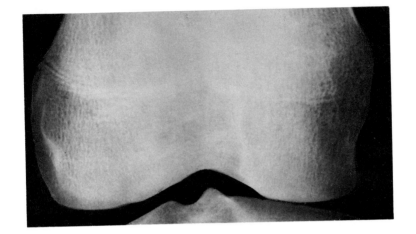

Grade 2

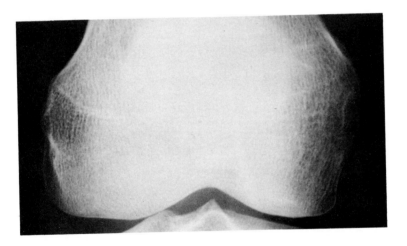

Grade 3

Figure 33.   Examples of FEM-L.

This is a very important indicator but it is
difficult to rate. If only a few trabeculae can be
traced from the metaphyseal area to the epiphyseal
area, in the anteroposterior view, this does not
necessarily indicate that some fusion is present.
This appearance may be due to the projection to a
single plane of trabeculae placed at different depths
(Fig. 34).

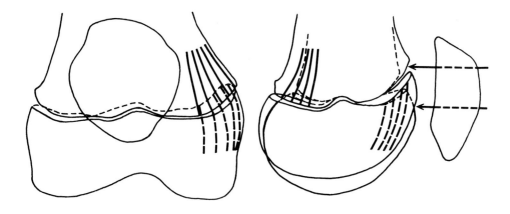

Figure 34. Diagrams of anteroposterior and lateral
radiographs showing how metaphyseal and epiphyseal
trabeculae at different depths can appear continuous
when projected to a single plane. This is relevant to
the grading of FEM-L, FEM-M, TIB-Q, TIB-R and FIB-F.

FEM-M

Medial epiphyseo-metaphyseal fusion: 3 grades

                                        Boys: 11 to 18 years
                                        Girls: 9 to 18 years

        Grade 1 -- absent

        Grade 2 -- incomplete

        Grade 3 -- complete

    This indicator refers to the part of the junction
medial to the indentation on the distal end of the
metaphysis (Fig. 35).

    The rules for assigning grades are the same as
for **FEM-L**.

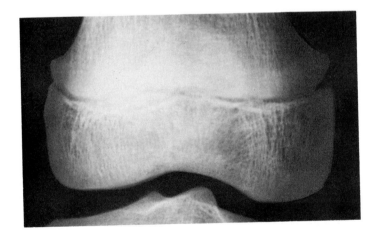

Figure 35.   FEM-M -- Grade 1.

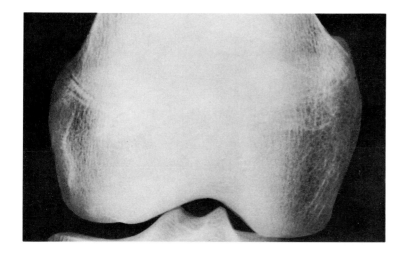

Grade 2

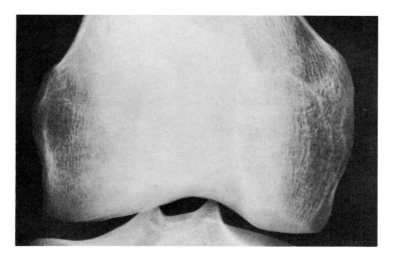

Grade 3

Figure 36.   Examples of FEM-M.

TIBIAL INDICATORS

The descriptions and age ranges are summarized in Table XX.   As for the femur, a ★ near the top of a page indicates that the plastic sheet (found in the back of this book) should be used.

TABLE XX

Summary of Indicators for Proximal End of Tibia

Indicator	Description	Grades	Age Range
TIB-A	Ratio EW/MW	5	Boys:1 mo.-10 yr. Girls:1 mo.-10 yr.
TIB-B	Ratio EW/EH	5	Boys:4.5-12 years Girls:3.5-12 yr.
TIB-C	Metaphyseal shape	2	Boys:1 mo.-1.5 yr. Girls:1 mo.-1.5 yr.
TIB-D	Epiphyseal shape	2	Boys:1 mo.-2 yr. Girls:1 mo.-1 yr.
TIB-E	Radio-opaque zone, lateral	2	Boys: 5-18 years Girls:3-18 years
TIB-F	Radio-opaque line, medial	2	Boys: 1-14 years Girls:1-16 years
TIB-G	Presence of tubercles	2	Boys:2.5-14 years Girls:1.5-12 yrs.
TIB-H	Height of tubercles	2	Boys: 7-18 years Girls:7-18 years
TIB-J	Shape of lateral intercondylar tubercle	2	Boys: 7-18 years Girls:7-18 years
TIB-K	Shape of medial intercondylar tubercle	2	Boys: 9-18 years Girls:6-18 years
TIB-L	Lateral epiphyseal margin	2	Boys: 1-10 years Girls:9 mo.-9 yr.
TIB-M	Lateral articular margin	2	Boys: 2.5-12 yr. Girls:2.5-9 yr.

(continued)

TABLE   XX   (continued)

Indicator	Description	Grades	Age range
TIB-N	Lateral capping	2	Boys:10-17 years Girls:8.5-16 yr.
TIB-P	Medial capping	2	Boys: 12-17 years Girls:9.5-17 yr.
TIB-Q	Lateral fusion	3	Boys: 12-18 years Girls:11-18 years
TIB-R	Medial fusion	3	Boys: 11-18 years Girls:11-18 years

TIB-A ★

Ratio $\dfrac{\text{epiphyseal width}}{\text{metaphyseal width}}$

Boys: 1 month to 10 years
Girls: 1 month to 10 years

TIB-A can be assessed only when an ossified epiphysis is present but fusion has not occurred. These measurements are made with a clear plastic rule to the nearest 0.5 mm.

The maximum width of the end of the metaphysis is measured, then the maximum width of the epiphysis is measured in the same plane used for the metaphysis (Fig. 37).

Areas of disseminated calcification are excluded but other irregularities of the margin are included.

This ratio should not be recorded in children with rickets.

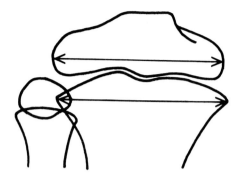

Figure 37. The planes in which epiphyseal and
metaphyseal widths of the tibia are measured.

TIB-B ★

Ratio $\dfrac{\text{epiphyseal width}}{\text{epiphyseal height}}$

                                    Boys: 4.5 to 12 years
                                    Girls: 3.5 to 12 years

        This measurement is made only if the metaphyseal
aspect of the epiphysis is flat (TIB-D; Grade 2) and
prior to fusion. Epiphyseal height is measured to the
nearest 0.5 mm as the maximum height <u>perpendicular</u> to
the plane in which the epiphyseal width is measured
(Fig. 38). The proximal end of the plane of measurement
is between the articular surfaces. A tubercle may be
included if the maximum plane passes through it.

        The epiphysis may project distally near the mid-
line. At younger ages, there may be a small projection
near the midline that is not superimposed on the
metaphysis. This is opposite to and curved reciprocally
with an indentation on the metaphysis. This small projection is included in the measurement. A second projection forms that becomes large, is superimposed on the
metaphysis and contributes to the formation of the tibial
tuberosity. It is <u>not</u> included in the measurement but
if the terminal plate of the epiphysis extends across
the prolongation the maximum height can be measured to
this part of the terminal plate (Fig. 38).

        The indicator cannot be assessed satisfactorily in
lower leg radiographs. It should not be recorded in
children with rickets.

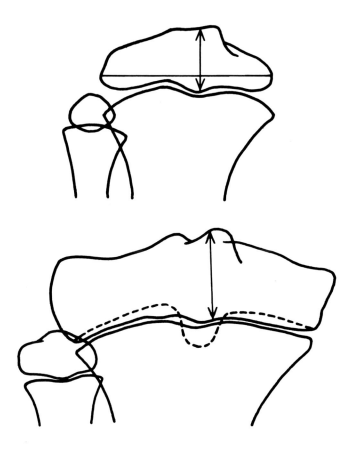

Figure 38. The plane in which epiphyseal height of
the tibia is measured (A) when there is no prolongation
of the epiphysis that is superimposed on the metaphysis
and (B) when such a prolongation is present.

                              TIB-C

Metaphyseal shape: 2 grades

                         Boys: 1 month to 1.5 years
                         Girls: 1 month to 1.5 years

         Grade 1 -- rounded or flattened

         Grade 2 -- indented

    This indicator, of course, cannot be assessed if
fusion has occurred.

    Grade 1 is assigned to radiographs in which the
epiphyseal aspect of the metaphysis is smoothly convex
proximally (Fig. 39). It is assigned also to radiographs in which the central part of this aspect is
flatter than the remainder.

    Grade 2 is recorded when this margin has an inden-
tation near the midline (Fig. 39).

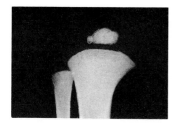

Grade 1
Rounded

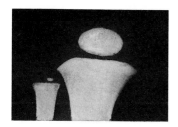

Grade 1
Flattened

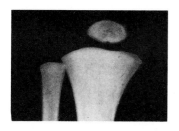

Grade 2
Slight

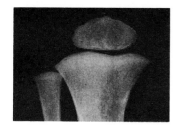

Grade 2
Moderate

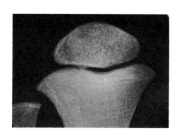

Grade 2
Marked

Figure 39.   Examples of TIB-C.

TIB-D

Flattening of metaphyseal aspect of the epiphysis:
                                                    2 grades

                                    Boys: 1 month to 2 years
                                    Girls: 1 month to 1 year

        Grade 1 -- absent

        Grade 2 -- present

        This indicator can be assessed only until fusion.
The margin of the epiphysis may be irregular particularly at younger ages (Fig. 40).

        Grade 1 is assigned when the epiphysis has not
ossified or when it is approximately elliptical or
ovoid. It is rarely circular but when this occurs
Grade 1 is assigned.

        Grade 2 is assigned when the epiphysis is flat on
part, but not necessarily all, of its metaphyseal
aspect. An epiphysis to which Grade 2 is assigned may
have a distal prolongation related to the indentation
on the end of the metaphysis.

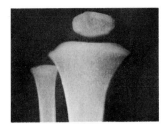

Grade 1

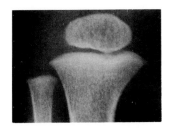

Grade 2
Slight

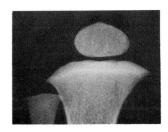

Grade 2
Irregular

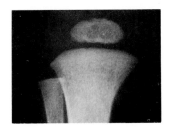

Grade 2
Irregular

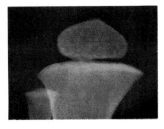

Grade 2
Marked

Figure 40.   Examples of TIB-D.

TIB-E

Radio-opaque zone due to the lateral articular surface:
                                                  2 grades

                                    Boys: 5 to 18 years
                                    Girls: 3 to 18 years

        Grade 1 -- absent

        Grade 2 -- present

    Usually this zone is distal to the midpart of the
lateral articular margin but it may appear on the
margin.

    For Grade 2 to be assigned, this zone must be
continuous and distinctly more radio-opaque than the
surrounding bony shadows. It must be wider than the
nearby trabeculae (Fig. 41).

    When there is slight lateral rotation of the knee,
this zone becomes less distinct but can still be
recognized.

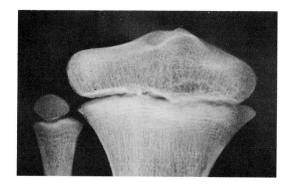

Grade 1

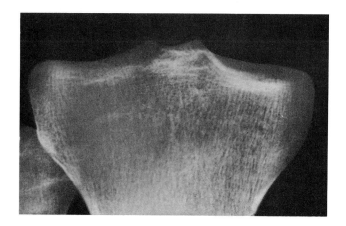

Grade 1
Discontinuous

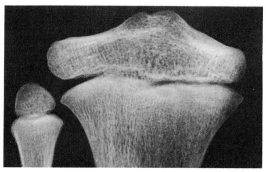

Grade 2

Figure 41.   Examples of TIB-E.

TIB-F

Radio-opaque line distal to the medial articular margin:
2 grades

Boys: 1 to 14 years
Girls: 1 to 16 years

Grade 1 -- absent

Grade 2 -- present

Grade 2 is assigned when there is a radio-opaque line <u>distal</u> to the medial articular margin. This line may extend into the area of the tubercles. The line must be thicker than the trabeculae and its proximal margin must be concave (Fig. 42).

TIB-F, unlike **TIB-E**, is referred to as a line, not a zone, because it has definite edges and it is narrow.

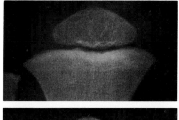

Grade 1
No radio-opaque line

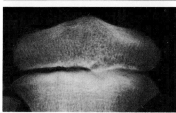

Grade 1
Radio-opaque zone but edges
    too indefinite for Grade 2

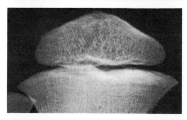

Grade 1
Line is on the margin, not
    distal to it

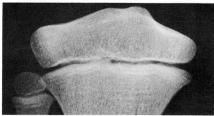

Grade 2
Line near the margin

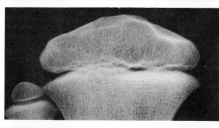

Grade 2

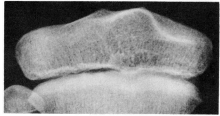

Grade 2
Line further from the margin

Figure 42.   Examples of TIB-F.

TIB-G

Tubercles between the medial and lateral articular
    surfaces: 2 grades

                                    Boys: 2.5 to 14 years
                                    Girls: 1.5 to 12 years

        Grade 1 -- absent

        Grade 2 -- present

    A tubercle is considered present when there is a
proximal projection from the margin of the epiphysis
between the medial and lateral articular surfaces.
Decisions regarding grades are based on the shape of
the margin between the lateral and medial articular
surfaces; radio-opaque lines within the epiphyseal
shadow are disregarded.

    Grade 1 is assigned when the junction between the
margins of the medial and lateral articular surfaces is
flat or only one tubercle is present, even if the flat
area is elevated as a plateau.

    Grade 2 is assigned when two tubercles project
proximally from the epiphysis (Fig. 43).

    This indicator cannot be assessed satisfactorily
in lower leg radiographs.

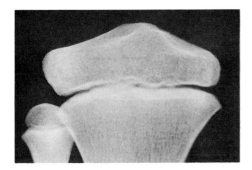

Grade 1
No tubercles

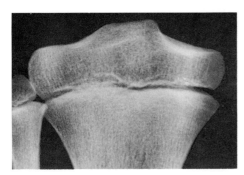

Grade 1
One tubercle

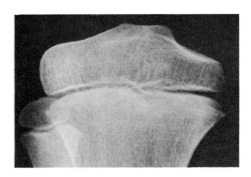

Grade 2
Two tubercles
Slight

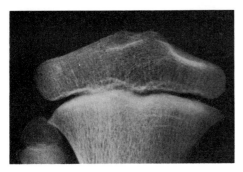

Grade 2
Two tubercles
Marked

Figure 43.   Examples of TIB-G.

TIB-H ★

Height of intercondylar tubercles: 2 grades

Boys: 7 to 18 years
Girls: 7 to 18 years

Grade 1 -- up to and including 2 mm

Grade 2 -- more than 2 mm

This is assessed only when tubercles are present (Tib-G; Grade 2). Grading is based on the distance, in the long axis of the tibia, from the apex of the taller tubercle to the lowest point in the indentation between the tubercles (Figs. 44 and 45).

This indicator cannot be graded satisfactorily in lower leg radiographs.

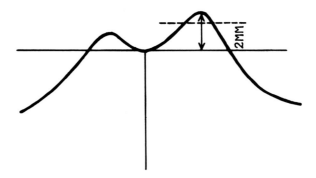

Figure 44. A diagram of the way in which the height of the tubercles is graded.

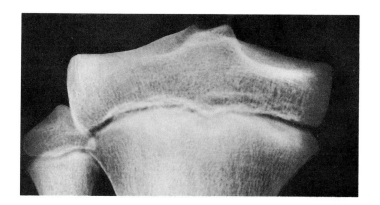

Grade 1

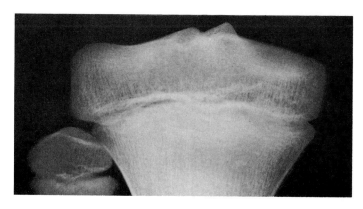

Grade 2

Figure 45.   Examples of TIB-H.

TIB-J ★

Shape of lateral intercondylar tubercle: 2 grades

                                    Boys: 7 to 18 years
                                    Girls: 7 to 18 years

Grade 1 -- flatter than Standard Curve V
          (7 mm long, major, 15 mm, $50°$)

Grade 2 -- more curved than, or as curved as,
          Standard Curve V

Grading is based on the shape of the margin; the radio-opaque line that may cross the tubercle is not used. The midpoint of the Standard Curve is fitted to the most pointed part of the margin of the tubercle keeping the Standard Curve aligned as in Figure 46.

In TIB-J and TIB-K the more mature grade is assigned to the more sharply curved margin.

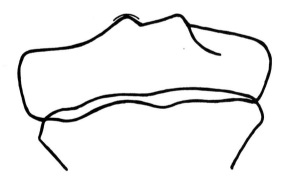

Figure 46. A diagram showing the part of the margin to which the standard curve is fitted.

Grade 1 is recorded if one or both ends of the Standard Curve are within the margin when the curve is fitted.

Grade 2 is assigned when the Standard Curve matches the margin or the ends of the curve lie outside the margin.

This indicator is sensitive to rotation of the knee in radiographic positioning. The presence of rotation is best judged from the radiographic position of the patella and the extent to which the shaft of the fibula is superimposed on that of the tibia.

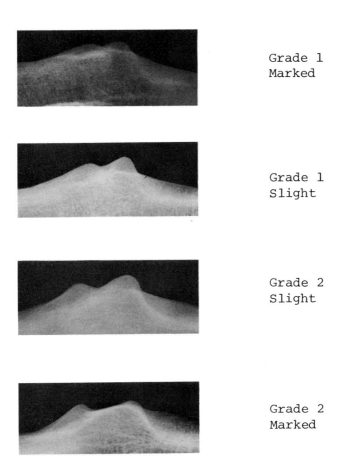

Grade 1
Marked

Grade 1
Slight

Grade 2
Slight

Grade 2
Marked

Figure 47.   Examples of TIB-J.

TIB-K ★

Shape of the medial intercondylar tubercle: 2 grades

                                        Boys: 9 to 18 years
                                        Girls: 6 to 18 years

            Grade 1 -- flatter than Standard Curve VI
                (7 mm long, major pole, 22 mm, 30°)

            Grade 2 -- equal to, or more curved than
                Standard Curve VI

        The Standard Curve is fitted in the same manner as
for TIB-J. The criteria for recording grades are the
same as in TIB-J but a different Standard Curve is used.
Examples of grades are shown in Figure 48.

        This indicator is sensitive to rotation in radio-
graphic positioning. As for TIB-J, the presence of
rotation is judged from the radiographic position of
the patella and the extent to which the shafts of the
tibia and fibula are superimposed. It cannot be
assessed satisfactorily in lower leg radiographs.

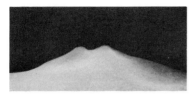

Grade 1

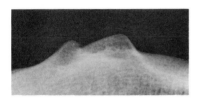

Grade 1

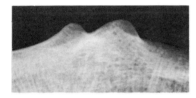

Grade 1

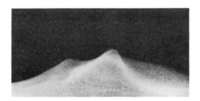

Grade 1
Grading must be based on the margin
  not the radio-opaque line

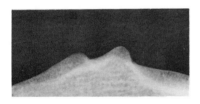

Grade 2

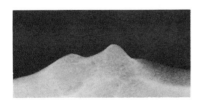

Grade 2

Figure 48.   Examples of grades of TIB-K.

TIB-L ★

Curvature of lateral nonarticular margin: 2 grades

Boys: 1 to 10 years
Girls: 9 months to 9 years

Grade 1 -- sharper than Standard Curve IV
(7 mm, major, 22 mm, 50°)

Grade 2 -- as curved or flatter than Standard
Curve IV (7 mm, major, 22 mm, 50°)

    The lateral nonarticular margin extends from the
lateral end of the articular surface to the lateral end
of the metaphyseal surface.   In relatively immature
children, these junctions are rounded: the lateral non-
articular margin is considered to extend to the mid-
points of these rounded areas.

    The Standard Curve is fitted to the central part
of the lateral nonarticular margin.   The area to which
the curve should be fitted is shown in Figure 49.
Examples of grades are shown in Figure 50.

    This indicator cannot be assessed satisfactorily
in lower leg radiographs.

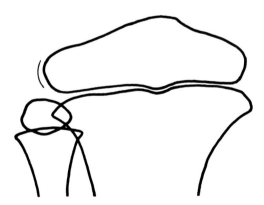

Figure 49.   The area to which the Standard Curve is
fitted in grading TIB-L.

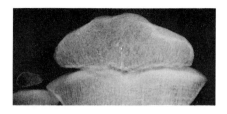

Grade 1
Marked

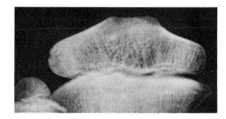

Grade 1
Slight

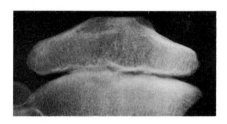

Grade 1
Irregular

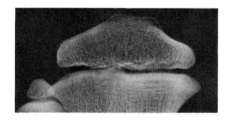

Grade 2
Slight

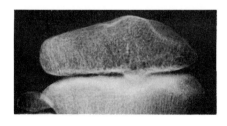

Grade 2
Marked

Figure 50.   Examples of TIB-L.

TIB-M ★

Curvature of lateral articular margin: 2 grades

Boys: 2.5 to 12 years
Girls: 2.5 to 9 years

Grade 1 -- convex or flat
Grade 2 -- concave

The area of the intercondylar eminence is omitted.
If this eminence has developed, it is excluded by plac-
ing a straight line along the lateral margin of the
lateral intercondylar tubercle and noting where this
margin begins to diverge from the line distally (Fig. 51).
Slight irregularities in the margin of the tubercle
are ignored.   The point of divergence defines the medial
end of the lateral articular margin.   A second line is
placed over the lateral articular margin from the above
point of divergence to the lateral proximal corner of
the epiphysis.   The indicator is graded by comparison
between the margin and this second line.   Grade 1 is
recorded if this comparison shows the margin is convex
or flat and Grade 2 if it is concave (Fig. 52). This
indicator cannot be assessed satisfactorily in lower leg
radiographs.

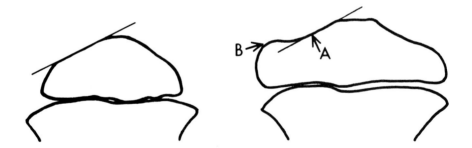

Figure 51. Diagrams of the area graded for TIB-M.
a. There is no intercondylar eminence; a straight line
has been placed on the lateral articular margin.
b. A straight line has been placed on the lateral margin
of the lateral intercondylar tubercle.   The margin
diverges from this line at the point of the arrow (A).
A second straight line is fitted from (A) to (B)--the
lateral proximal corner of the epiphysis.

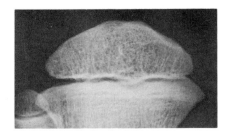

Grade 1
Convex

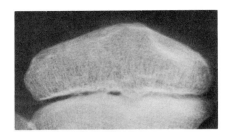

Grade 1
Flat, without an eminence

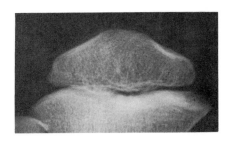

Grade 1
Flat, with an eminence

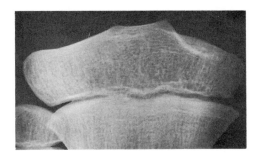

Grade 2

Figure 52.   Examples of TIB-M.

TIB-N

Capping at lateral end of epiphyseo-metaphyseal junction:
                                                2 grades

                                  Boys: 10 to 17 years
                                  Girls: 8.5 to 16 years

        Grade 1 -- absent

        Grade 2 -- present

    Corresponding criteria are used for TIB-N and
TIB-P. These indicators refer to capping on the
lateral and medial ends of the epiphyseo-metaphyseal
junction respectively.

    Grade 2 is recorded if the junction between the
nonarticular and the distal margins of the epiphysis
is pointed and directed distally (Fig. 53).

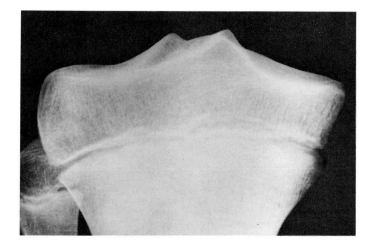

Grade 1

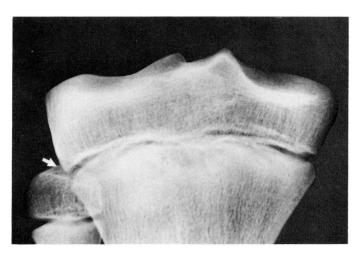

Grade 2

Figure 53.   Examples of TIB-N.

TIB-P

Capping at medial end of epiphyseo-metaphyseal junction:
2 grades

Boys: 12 to 17 years
Girls: 9.5 to 17 years

Grade 1 -- absent

Grade 2 -- present

The criteria used are the same as those described for TIB-N. Examples of grades are shown in Figure 54.

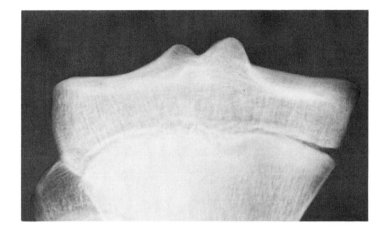

Grade 1

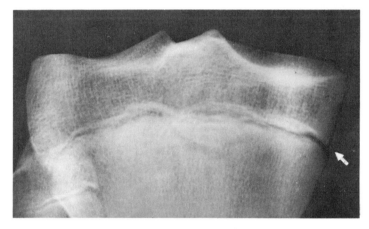

Grade 2

Figure 54.   Examples of TIB-P.

TIB-Q

Fusion in the lateral part of the epiphyseo-metaphyseal
        junction: 3 grades

                                    Boys: 12 to 18 years
                                    Girls: 11 to 18 years

        Grade 1 -- absent

        Grade 2 -- incomplete

        Grade 3 -- complete

        The part of the junction near the midline (about
half the total width) is obscured by the tibial
tuberosity and is not graded in TIB-Q or TIB-R.   The
areas inspected when these indicators are graded are
shown in Figure 55.

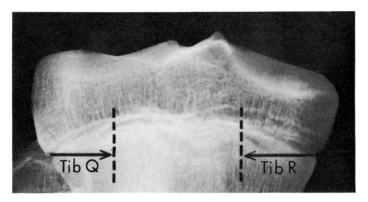

Figure 55.   The areas assessed in TIB-Q and TIB-R.

Grade 1 is assigned when the lateral part of the junction is a relatively radiolucent strip or consists of several discontinuous strips that overlap and collectively extend for the whole length of the area considered (Fig. 56).

Grade 2 is recorded when definite bony fusion is present across part but not all of the lateral part of the junction (Fig. 57). If a few trabeculae can be traced from the metaphyseal area to the epiphyseal area, this does not necessarily indicate that some fusion is present. This appearance may be due to the projection, to a single plane, of trabeculae at different depths, as shown in Figure 34 for FEM-L. The best evidence of fusion is the absence of a radiolucent epiphyseal zone.

Grade 3 is assigned when fusion is complete or if only a notch remains in the cortical margin. After fusion is complete, a radio-opaque line may persist at the level where fusion occurred.

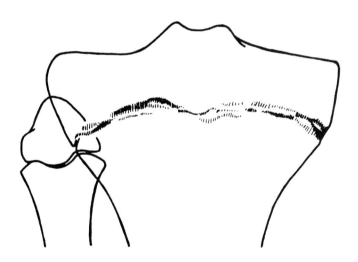

Figure 56. A diagram showing discontinuous radiolucent strips that collectively extend for the whole length of the epiphyseo-metaphyseal junction (Grade 1, TIB-Q and TIB-R).

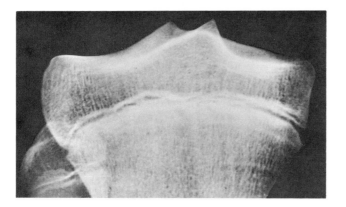

Grade 1

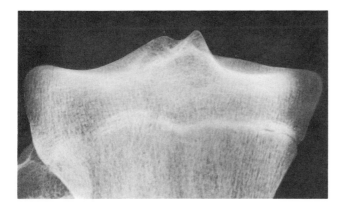

Grade 2

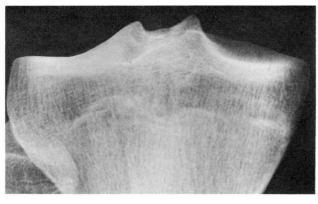

Grade 3

Figure 57.   Examples of TIB-Q.

FIBULAR INDICATORS

The descriptions and age ranges are summarized in Table XXI. As before, a ★ near the top of a page shows that the plastic sheet at the back of the book should be used.

TABLE   XXI

Summary of Indicators for Proximal End of Fibula

Indicator Description	Grades	Age range
FIB-A Ratio EW/MW	5	Boys: 3.5 to 16 years Girls: 3 to 14 years
FIB-B Metaphyseal shape	2	Boys: 1 to 9 years Girls: 3 months to 7 years
FIB-C Epiphyseal shape	3	Boys: 1 to 9 years Girls: 1 to 7 years
FIB-D Terminal plate	2	Boys: 3.5 to 15 years Girls: 2 to 14 years
FIB-E Styloid process	2	Boys: 7 to 16 years Girls: 6 to 14 years
FIB-F Fusion	4	Boys: 11 to 18 years Girls: 10 to 18 years

FIB-A ★

Ratio $\dfrac{\text{epiphyseal width}}{\text{metaphyseal width}}$

Boys: 3.5 to 16 years
Girls: 3 to 14 years

FIB-A can be assessed only when an ossified epiphysis is present but fusion has not occurred. Metaphyseal width is measured as the maximum diameter, to the nearest 0.5 mm; the maximum epiphyseal width is measured in the same plane as metaphyseal width (Fig. 59).

At later ages, this indicator cannot be recorded in some radiographs because the proximal end of the fibula is superimposed on an increasingly opaque tibia.

This ratio should not be recorded in children with rickets.

Figure 59. The planes in which the epiphyseal and metaphyseal width of the fibula are measured.

FIB-B

Shape of the proximal margin of the metaphysis: 2 grades

Boys: 1 to 9 years
Girls: 3 months to 7 years

Grade 1 -- concave, convex or flat

Grade 2 -- indented

Whenever possible, assessment is based on the
thick radio-opaque line usually present at the proximal
end of the metaphysis. If this line is not present
the margin is used. This indicator cannot be assessed
after fusion nor in radiographs in which the margin
is superimposed on the epiphysis.

Grade 1 is assigned when the metaphyseal margin
is flat or convex or when the whole margin is concave.
A concave margin was very unusual and occurred only
during the first few months of life (Fig. 60).

Grade 2 is assigned when only part of the margin
is indented, usually near the midline of the bone.
Even when large, the indentation does not extend as
far as both margins.

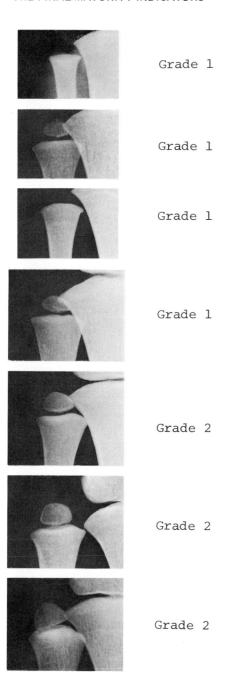

Grade 1

Grade 1

Grade 1

Grade 1

Grade 2

Grade 2

Grade 2

Figure 60.   Examples of FIB-B.

FIB-C ★

Epiphyseal shape: 3 grades

                                                    Boys: 1 to 9 years
                                                    Girls: 1 to 7 years

        Grade 1 -- not ossified

        Grade 2 -- metaphyseal margin is convex

        Grade 3 -- metaphyseal margin is flattened

        This indicator can be assessed only when fusion
has not occurred.

        Grade 2 is recorded if the metaphyseal margin of
the epiphysis is convex. The general shape of the
epiphysis, e.g., round, elliptical, ovoid, is not used
as a basis for grading (Figs. 61-62).

        Grade 3 is assigned if the metaphyseal margin is
generally flat. Recognition of flattening of the
metaphyseal margin is assisted by using the line at
which the maximum width of the epiphysis is measured
and comparing the curvatures of the margins proximal
and distal to this. The presence of a slight distal
projection from the metaphyseal margin does not prevent
the assignment of Grade 3 (Fig. 62). Rarely, the
epiphysis may have two centers; when this occurs it
cannot be graded.

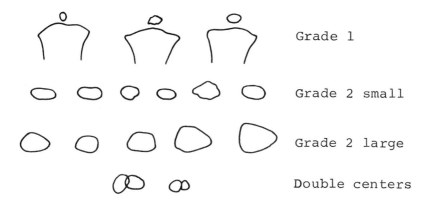

Grade 1

Grade 2 small

Grade 2 large

Double centers

Figure 61. A diagram showing the range of variation
in shape to which grades of FIB-C were assigned,
together with examples of double centers.

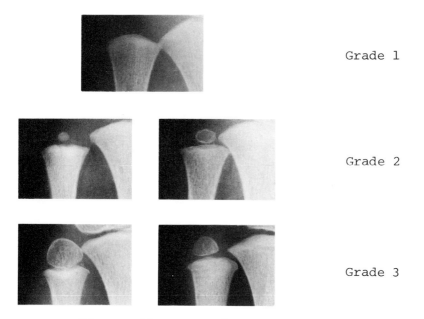

Grade 1

Grade 2

Grade 3

Figure 62. Examples of FIB-C.

FIB-D

Terminal plate: 2 grades

                                    Boys: 3.5 to 15 years
                                    Girls: 2 to 14 years

          Grade 1 -- absent

          Grade 2 -- present

       This indicator cannot be assessed after fusion
has occurred.

       Grade 2 is assigned when there is a dense radio-
opaque line on at least half the length of the
metaphyseal margin of the epiphysis (Fig. 63).

       Due to obliquity of the epiphyseal zone, the edge
of the metaphyseal margin of the epiphysis may be
visible as an ellipse (Fig. 64).

       If the epiphyseal and metaphyseal shadows are
superimposed and a dense radio-opaque line is present
both within and beyond the area of superimposition, the
whole line is considered a terminal plate (Grade 2).
If, however, a radio-opaque line is present only in
the area of superimposition, this indicator is not
graded because one cannot be certain that this line is
due to a terminal plate.

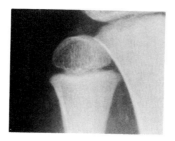

Grade 1

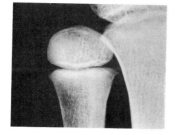

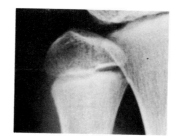

Grade 2

Grade 2
Partly superimposed

Figure 63.   Examples of FIB-D.

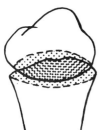

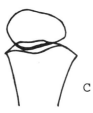

A   B   C

Figure 64.   Diagrams of the epiphyseo-metaphyseal area
of the fibula.   A. The adjoining surfaces of the
epiphysis and metaphysis appear elliptical and they are
partially superimposed.   B. The heavy line shows the
possible position of a terminal plate (Grade 2).
C. Radio-opaque line present only in the area of
superimposition (not graded).

FIB-E

Styloid process: 2 grades

                                    Boys: 7 to 16 years
                                    Girls: 6 to 14 years

            Grade 1 -- absent

            Grade 2 -- present

    Grade 2 is assigned when there is a projection
from the proximal margin of the epiphysis (Fig. 65).
Usually this is on the medial side but it may appear
centrally or laterally placed due to variations in
radiographic positioning.

    When the styloid process is centrally or laterally
placed, Grade 2 is not assigned unless a radio-opaque
line or zone crosses the epiphysis and the projection
extends further proximally than the most proximal part
of the line or zone.

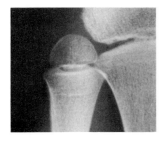

Grade 1

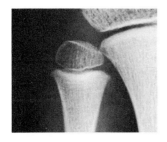

Grade 1 with radio-opaque line

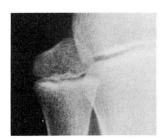

Grade 2 with process placed medially

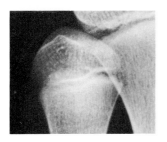

Grade 2 with process placed laterally

Figure 65. Examples of FIB-E.

FIB-F

Fusion of the epiphyseal-metaphyseal junction: 4 grades

                                    Boys: 11 to 18 years
                                    Girls: 10 to 18 years

        Grade 1 -- absent

        Grade 2 -- incomplete

        Grade 3 -- complete except for a notch at one
                   or both cortical margins

        Grade 4 -- complete

   Assessment is based on the part of the zone not
superimposed on the tibia. The epiphyseal zone is
oblique anteroposteriorly and it may have a double
radiographic image.

   Grade 1 is assigned when the junction is a
relatively radiolucent strip or consists of several
discontinuous strips that overlap and collectively
extend for the whole distance considered (Fig. 66).

   Grade 2 is recorded when definite bony fusion is
present across part but not all of the junction. If
a few trabeculae can be traced from the metaphyseal
area to the epiphyseal area, this does not necessarily
indicate some fusion is present. This appearance may
be due to the projection, to a single plane, of
trabeculae at different depths, as shown in Figure 34
for FEM-L. The best evidence of fusion is the absence
of a radiolucent epiphyseal zone.

   Grade 3 is assigned when fusion is complete
throughout the area considered but a radiolucent notch
still remains in one or both cortical margins.

   Grade 4 is recorded when fusion is complete.
A radio-opaque line may still be present at the level
of fusion.

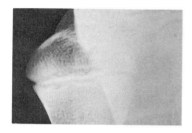

Grade 1
Continuous gap

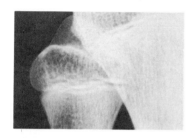

Grade 1
Discontinuous gap

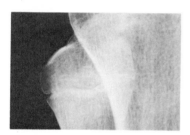

Grade 2

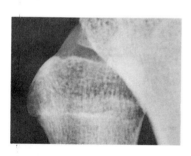

Grade 3

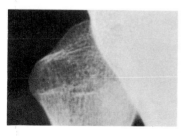

Grade 4

Figure 66.   Examples of FIB-F.

CHAPTER   V

THE STATISTICAL BASIS OF THE SCORING METHOD

The Problem

Traditionally the concept of skeletal age has been associated with the idea that there are individual differences in the rate of maturation. Variations among individuals in skeletal age (SA) at any given chronological age (CA) reflects this differential rate of previous maturation. But, at the same time, across individuals of a given CA, the average SA should be the same as that CA. This suggests a particular approach to the calibration of an assessment scheme for SA in which the problem is taken to be one of prediction, the dependent variable is CA (across ages), and the independent variables (the predictor variables) are, in the present case, the various maturity indicators described in Chapter IV. Thus, it is assumed that there is a variable, skeletal maturity, that is related linearly to CA across ages, and the aim is to estimate skeletal maturity from the pattern of maturity as observed in a complex set of indicators within a single radiograph.

The problem is to form an index from these indicators that predicts CA across age with maximal accuracy. The variance of estimated skeletal maturity within CA is interpreted as a combination of what has been classically referred to as the variance of SA and error variance. The separation of the within age variance into these two components has been impossible with prior methodologies, except by assuming that the only error is in scorer unreliability and using inter- and

intra-rater reliabilities to estimate this error.
This is unsatisfactory, because inter- and intra-rater
variance represents only part of the true error variance.

Before approaching a possible solution, it is
often helpful to consider the properties of an optimal
solution; then the possible solution can be compared
with the ideal. First we want a method that can estimate SA for every person at every CA between the two
extremes of complete immaturity and full maturity.
These estimates should employ all the available items
of information, weighting them differentially depending on their reliability and usefulness. When the
recorded maturity indicators yield insufficient information to provide accurate estimates of SA, the method
should tell us so, and in addition, should give a
measure of accuracy for each estimate. In fact, it
should be possible to obtain stochastic confidence
intervals around each estimate. The estimates them-
selves should be scaled in a reasonable way, and
"year" would be the most natural "unit" for this
purpose. The estimates should have a number of statistically desirable characteristics, such as,
asymptotic efficiency and minimum sufficiency.
Summarizing these characteristics in more common
terminology, the method should use whatever information is available in the data as fully and efficiently
as possible.

To add to what is already a long list of requirements for an optimal solution, let us include that
missing data be allowed (that is, an estimate should
be possible for an individual even if some desirable
data are missing), and that the model allow use of a
subset of predictor variables and do the best it can
with what is available. Finally, to assist future
research workers, the method should allow the addition
of other variables (maturity indicators that are not
currently available) without serious modification or
renorming of the method. These could be other types
of variables or similar variables from other parts of
the skeleton. It seems impossible to meet all these
requirements, particularly when the available data

are not carefully measured ratio scaled variables, but
a mixture of grades assigned to each of a large number
of indicators. The task, however, is not impossible.

A Solution

During the last two decades, several statisticians
and psychometricians have worked on the development of
a class of models that exactly fills the needs stated
previously. The earliest of these models (Lazarsfeld,
1959) contained only the germ of what was to come, but
Lazarsfeld expanded his own work (Lazarsfeld and Henry,
1968) and important contributions were made by others
(e.g., Birnbaum, 1968; Samejima, 1969; Bock, 1972).
What has resulted from this work will be described in
the next section of this chapter in elementary terms
and in the following section in precise detail. Those
who wish, will find an opaque, though fully explicated,
version in Samejima's (1969) original monograph.

The model that has been used has the following
characteristics:

(a) It uses graded category scoring to obtain
interval estimates of maturity.

(b) using the method of maximum likelihood, these
estimates have most of the generally desirable statistical qualities[*], in that asymptotically they make

---

[*] They are not unbiased, which is a minor deficit, and
they have some other statistical peculiarities in this
context to which Berkson (1955) has directed attention. Namely, because they are sufficient statistics,
they do not allow improvement through Rao-Blackwell-
ization. Berkson argues convincingly that, for small
samples (N less than 10), improved minimum logit chi-
square estimates are better than maximum likelihood
estimates though substantially more difficult to com-
pute. This is marginally applicable in the present
case because Berkson's use of the logistic model in
bio-assay is very similar to the one proposed here.

maximal use of the available information.

(c) It provides standard errors for these estimates, so that the within CA variance of maturity
estimates can be decomposed to two components: (i) the
variance due to differences between maturity levels and
(ii) the variance due to error.

(d) The scale and unit of measurement is arbitrary.
Hence, use of the natural "year" scale is accomplished
easily by scaling so that the means and variances of the
obtained SA estimates are the same as the means and
variances of CA in the sample.

(e) A most important reason for utilizing a latent
trait model (paraphrasing Bock and Wood, 1971) in the
assessment of maturity is that, given this set of cali-
brated indicators, that we will show fit the latent
trait model, maturity scores can be calculated on the
same scale from ratings on any subset of indicators.
This means, in particular, that alternate or partial
forms of the method may be scored on a common scale
without resorting to renorming, and that comparable
scores can be obtained when, as often happens, not all
indicators are available for each subject. In addition,
the model allows the rigorous implementation of sequential assessments in which, at any state of assessment,
a maturity score and its associated error of measurement
can be ascertained. Thus, in a computer assisted situation, an additional indicator can be selected that will
yield maximum benefit in regard to increased accuracy,
and the scheme can stop as soon as the standard error of
the maturity estimate becomes acceptably small. This
is very important because, as we shall see, the individual indicators are differentially helpful at various
levels of maturity. Thus one can use a reasonable
guess (prompted by CA and sex) to determine a first
group of indicators that can yield a preliminary maturity estimate. Subsequently, additional indicators
known to be useful at that maturity level could be
scored. This process can be repeated yielding refined
estimates of maturity until a satisfactory level of
accuracy has been attained.

(f) In addition, the latent trait model has the advantage of measurement on a scale with a well-defined metric. This means that skeletal maturity estimates, or any allowable transformation of them that theory may dictate, can be used to measure changes in levels and rates of skeletal maturation. This is particularly important if the purpose is to evaluate the efficacy of intervention programs. Traditional methods of maturity assessment are markedly deficient in this respect and have hindered the study of change.

(g) The latent trait model allows the addition of other indicators (e.g., in the hand-wrist) by simply calibrating each new indicator to CA. Thus it becomes easy to build upon the present system for the knee joint and to further reduce the error, that is increase the accuracy. There is no unnecessary irradiation, because the information in one radiograph is utilized fully before another radiograph is taken to achieve greater accuracy, should that be needed. This is a great advantage and it implies that the latent trait method yields a common system by which research workers can weigh the respective usefulness of various sites and indicators.

The Latent Trait Model

Having outlined the efficacy of latent trait models, we shall describe the nature of these models and how they work. To avoid unnecessary complication, the simplest case will be described, that for binary indicators. Among the 34 maturity indicators for the knee, 19 are of this type.

The model posits a unidimensional latent space, i.e., a single latent variable, skeletal maturity, the effects of which are observable on a number of manifest variables (maturity indicators). These indicators, through their degree of development in the radiograph, can be categorized with respect to their degree of maturity. A precise technical description of the analytic model is found in the original source (Samejima, 1969). What follows is a heuristic, intuitive and

sometimes slightly inaccurate description. It is hoped
that this will, however, allow the reader to understand
the results presented here.

We will first describe the model for binary indicators: indicators with only two grades, mature and
immature. For each indicator at each CA, the proportion of the sample that is mature is computed. The
type of data obtained is shown in Figure 67. A logistic function is fitted to these observed proportions
as a function of CA.

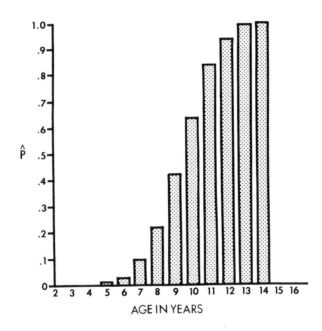

Figure 67. Proportions of individuals at various chronological ages that are mature on indicator j (denoted $\hat{P}_j$).

This is shown in equation (1),

(1) $\hat{P}_j = \{1 + \exp(-d_j [T_j + CA])\}^{-1}$

where
$\hat{P}_j$ = the observed proportion of individuals mature
     on indicator j,

CA = chronological age,

T_j = the chronological age at which 50 percent of
    the sample are mature for this indicator
    (the so-called "threshold") and

d_j = the discriminability (slope) of this indicator
    that reflects its rate of maturation.

This is very similar to probit analysis that is used
widely in bio-assay and in studies of growth and maturation (Hogben et al., 1948; Tanner et al., 1972, 1975;
Aitchison and Silvey, 1967). The difference is in the
use of a logistic rather than the Normal ogive function
to fit the proportions. In practice, the logistic is
practically indistinguishable from the Normal ogive, but
mathematically the logistic is the more tractable of the
two. For this reason and others (see Berkson, 1951),
the logistic has been used in the current application.

A logistic function fitted to the data given in
Figure 67 is shown in Figure 68. The estimated proportion obtained from the fitted function is interpreted
as the probability that a person of a particular CA will
have indicator j mature. This probability is denoted P_j.

Note that different indicators can have the same
slope (d) but different values of T (the "threshold").
This implies these indicators have equal discriminating
power, but they are applicable at different chronological ages and thus at different stages of development.
Three such indicators are shown in Figure 69.

Conversely, several indicators can have the same
value of T but different discriminating abilities. In
general, the steeper the slope, the more discriminating

the indicator in regard to maturity. Figure 70
includes the curves (probability of being mature) for
two indicators having different values of d but the
same threshold.

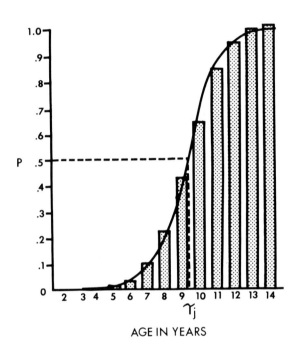

Figure 68. A fitted logistic function to the observed
proportions of individuals at various chronological
ages who are mature on indicator j.

Summarizing, for each indicator j, there is a representation of maturation as a three parameter logistic function, and the probability of an indicator being mature for a particular skeletal age θ is:

$$(2) \qquad P_j \ (x_j = 2 | \ \theta) \ = \ \{1 + \exp[-d_j \ (T_j + \theta)] \ \}^{-1}$$

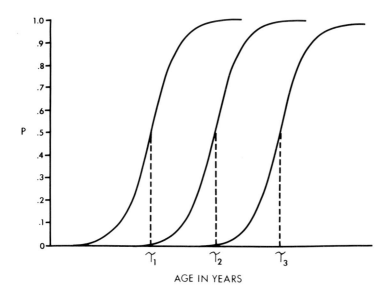

AGE IN YEARS

Figure 69. An example of three indicators (1, 2 and 3) having the same slope (discriminating ability) but different thresholds (T_1, T_2 and T_3).

where $x_j = \begin{cases} 1 \text{ if indicator j is not mature} \\ 2 \text{ if indicator j is mature,} \end{cases}$

d_j = the slope of the fitted logistic associated with indicator j,

T_j = the threshold (50 percent point) for indicator j and

Θ = SA.

Note, of course, that

$$P_j (x_j = 1| \Theta) = 1 - P_j (x_j = 2| \Theta).$$

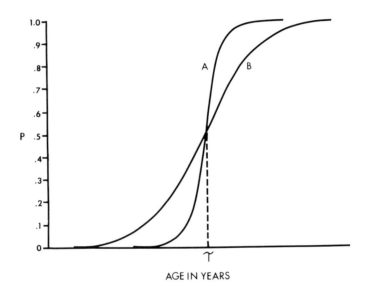

AGE IN YEARS

Figure 70. An example of two indicators that have the same threshold but different slopes. B is less discriminatory than A and so is less useful as a maturity indicator.

It is important to explicate fully a crucial intuitive step. Up to this point, the parameters for each indicator were integrally tied to CA, in that logistic functions were fitted to the proportions of the sample in which each indicator was mature at each CA. Once these parameters are established, the obverse question is asked: "Given the observed pattern of maturity indicators, what is the most likely CA of the person having this pattern?" This estimate of CA, obtained from maturity indicators, is called SA and is denoted θ.

The steps followed in obtaining this estimate are as follows:

(a) Estimate the indicator parameters from equation (1).

(b) Using methods to be described shortly, determine the value of θ that maximizes the probability of the observed pattern of x_j's. The observed pattern of x_j's for n indicators is denoted by $\underline{x}$, a vector of length n.

To do this, the probability of a particular pattern is represented by the product of the probabilities of each of the indicators. This product is shown in equation (3).

(3)
$$P(\underline{x}\mid\theta) = \prod_{j=1}^{n} P_j(x_j\mid\theta).$$

For this representation to hold, the various values of P_j must be conditionally independent, given θ. This has been assumed to be the case. The preceding description refers to the model for a series of binary indicators; the more general case for indicators with multiple grades is similar and is described in detail in the next section.

distributed as Chi-square and hence we can use (6) to
test for a significant departure from fit.

(6)
$$X^2_j = \sum_{i=1}^{k} \; n_i \; \frac{(\hat{P}_{ij} - P_{ij})^2}{P_{ij}}$$

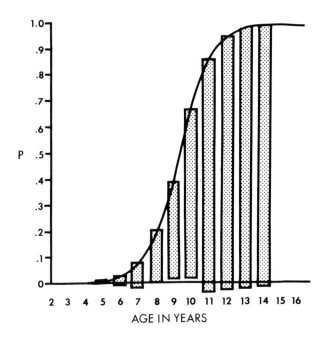

Figure 71. Hanging histogram of observed proportions
of individuals at various chronological ages who are
mature on indicator j hung from logistic function
describing the relationship between maturity on j and
chronological age.

where the data are examined at k different ages. We sum over all of them and

n_i = number of individuals who were evaluated at age i,

P_{ij} = the logistically fitted estimate of the proportion of individuals in whom indicator j was mature when they were in age group i and

$\hat{P}_{ij}$ = the observed proportion of individuals in whom indicator j was mature when they were in age group i.

Thus we can determine the extent and significance of any departure from fit. Proceeding in a similar fashion, and making the assumption of normally distributed error, we can use the error term obtained from the second derivative of equation (3) to construct a stochastic confidence bound around the estimates of θ. This allows us to determine within what range of values a particular individual's true SA falls with any specified degree of accuracy. No other existing method can do this.

The Graded Case

Previously the observed data were denoted by the vector of length n, $\underline{x}$, in which the entries of $\underline{x}$ were $x_j = \begin{cases} 1 \\ 2 \end{cases}$ where 1 is assigned if indicator j is immature and 2 if it is mature.

The multiple graded case assumes that each indicator can be graded from 1 to m_j, where m_j is the maximum grade and represents the complete level of maturity of indicator j. For the binary case $m_j = 2$, but m_j can vary from indicator to indicator. Thus we now define the response vector in the graded case to be $\underline{v}$, where $\underline{v}' = (v_1, v_2, \ldots, v_n)$ and each v_j can take grades $1, 2, \ldots, m_j$. The greater the value of v_j, the greater the maturity of the j indicator.

The model representing the functional relationship between the proportion mature and skeletal age is slightly more complex for the general graded case than for the binary case. It is

$$(7) \quad P(v_j = \ell \mid \theta) = \{1 + \exp[-d_j(T_{j, \ell-1} + \theta)]\}^{-1} -$$
$$\{1 + \exp[-d_j(T_{j\ell} - \theta)]\}^{-1}$$
$$= p_{j, \ell-1} - p_{j\ell}, \text{ where } p_{j0} = 1 \text{ and } p_{jm_j} = 0.$$

Note that $p_{j, \ell-1}$ is the cumulative probability that an individual of maturity θ is assigned grade ℓ or some more mature grade $(\ell+1, \ell+2, \text{ etc.})$, and $p_{j\ell}$ is the cumulative probability that the individual is assigned a more mature grade than ℓ. Thus, equation (7), the difference between $p_{j, \ell-1}$ and $p_{j\ell}$ is $P(V_j = \ell \mid \theta)$, the probability that an individual of maturity θ will be graded ℓ on indicator j. Probability curves for the general graded curve are in Figure 72 for $m_j = 3$. Note several differences between this figure and Figure 68. Figure 68 displays only $P(v_j = 2)$ because there were only two grades and one is the complement of the other. In the current situation,

$$P(v_j = 1) = 1 - P(v_j = 2) - P(v_j = 3);$$

consequently it is better to display all curves. Samejima (1969) calls these "operating characteristic" curves. The first curve $P(v_j = 1)$ shows that at low θ

(marked immaturity) all individuals are in this class; in other words, everyone is graded "1" for indicator j. As maturity progresses (θ increases; greater skeletal age), individuals move into grade 2 so the curve $P(v_j = 2)$ increases with a corresponding decrease in $P(v_j = 1)$. This continues until virtually everyone is or has been in this category (grade 2). As later

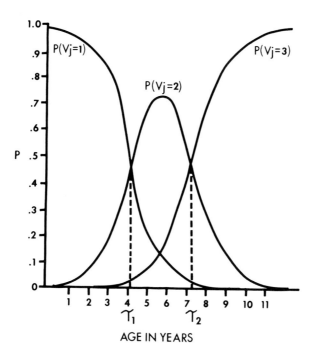

Figure 72. An illustrative set of operating character-istic curves for the case of three ordered grades.

chronological ages are considered, the indicator matures further and is scored "grade 3," thus the $P(v_j = 2)$ curve decreases and the $P(v_j = 3)$ curve increases.

For indicators with more than three grades, the picture is similar, but more complex. With four grades, there are two bell-shaped curves between the two ogives; with five grades, three bell-shaped curves between the ogives. However, even in the more complex cases, the thresholds still fall at 50 percent, that is at T_1, 50 percent are scored "grade 1" and 50 percent are "grade 2" or "grade 3": at T_2, 50 percent are scored "grade 3" and 50 percent are scored "grade 1" or "grade 2."

The Latent Trait Model for the Multiple Graded Case

This technical section is adapted from Kolakowski and Bock (1973). For mathematical simplicity, it is necessary to modify the earlier presentation in specifying the general model. Therefore let us define, as before:

$j = 1, 2, \ldots, n$ indicators, each scored in m_j ordered categories, with category 1 the least mature. Next we introduce a modest notational change and allow the data for each subject to be represented as a matrix R having elements $\{r_{jk}\}$, where

$$r_{jk} = \begin{cases} 1 \text{ if indicator } j \text{ is scored in category } k \\ 0 \text{ if scored otherwise,} \end{cases}$$

θ = the skeletal age for a given subject and

P_{jk} = the probability that $r_{jk} = 1$

$$P_{jk} = \left\{1 + \exp[-d_j (T_{j,k-1} - \theta)]\right\}^{-1} - \left\{1 + \exp[-d_j (T_{jk} - \theta)]\right\}^{-1}$$

$$P_{jk} = P_{j,k-1} - P_{jk}$$

where $p_{jo} = 1$ and $p_{jm_j} = 0$.   Then

$$P(R|\theta) = \prod_{j=1}^{n} \prod_{k=1}^{m_j} P_{jk}^{r_{jk}}$$

Thus it follows that the likelihood function of θ is

$$L(\theta|R) = \prod_{j=1}^{n} \prod_{k=1}^{m_j} P_{jk}^{r_{jk}}$$

Therefore a log transformation yields

$$C = \log L(\theta|R) = \sum_{j}^{n} \sum_{k}^{m_j} r_{jk} \log P_{jk}$$

which will again be used to assist calculation.

Taking derivitives gives

$$\frac{\partial C}{\partial \theta} = \sum_j \sum_k \frac{r_{jk}}{P_{jk}} \frac{\partial P_{jk}}{\partial \theta} = \sum_j \sum_k \frac{r_{jk} d_j (P_{j,k-1}q_{j,k-1} - P_{jk}q_{jk})}{P_{jk}}$$

where $q_{jk} = 1 - P_{jk}$;

$$\frac{\partial^2 C}{\partial \theta^2} = \sum_j \sum_k \left[\frac{r_{jk}}{P_{jk}} \frac{\partial^2 P_{jk}}{\partial \theta^2} - \frac{r_{jk}}{P_{jk}} \left(\frac{\partial P_{jk}}{\partial \theta} \right)^2 \right]$$

$$= \sum_j d_j^2 \sum_k \frac{r_{jk}}{P_{jk}} \left[(q_{j,k-1} - P_{j,k-1}) P_{j,k-1}q_{j,k-1} \right.$$

$$+ (p_{jk} - q_{jk}) P_{jk}q_{jk}$$

$$\left. - \frac{(P_{jk}q_{jk} - P_{j,k-1}q_{j,k-1})^2}{P_{jk}} \right]$$

Using the Newton-Raphson method to any g^{th} stage estimate of θ yields,

$$\theta_{g+1} = \theta_g - \frac{\partial C}{\partial \theta} \bigg/ \frac{\partial^2 C}{\partial \theta^2} .$$

The statistical model, as described, appears, on the surface, to offer hope for the development of an objective scheme for the assessment of skeletal maturity. Although a model has been specified and an estimation scheme for determining its parameters developed, one cannot be certain of its efficacy until it is tested. The model could be inappropriate; in which case it would not account adequately for the observed data. Another problem could be the accurate specification of the parameters; the standard errors could be so large that the assessment is worthless. As will be shown shortly, these worries are groundless. The method converges well and estimates skeletal age in situations when other methods fail. In short, it ful-fills in practice all the criteria specified for an optimal solution.

THE GRADING OF THE RATIO INDICATORS

Twenty-eight of the indicators described in Chapter IV yield measurements in the form of ordered grades. Consequently, the analytical model just described is directly applicable. Six of the indicators, FEM-A, FEM-B, FEM-C, TIB-A, TIB-B, and FIB-A, yield measurements in the form of ratios, and so do not directly fit the requirements of the analytical model. However, it is simple to solve this problem without losing any of the advantages of the latent trait model. The solution is to make the ratio indicators into graded indicators. To achieve this end, five grades (numbered 1 through 5) are established for each of the six ratio indicators, and ratio values for each indi-cator are assigned to grades depending on whether they lie between fixed boundary values.

The boundary values for the grading of the ratio indicators are given in Table XXII.   There are four boundary values for each indicator, denoted Boundary (1) through Boundary (4).   In all cases, Boundary (0) = 0 and Boundary (5) = ∞.   A ratio indicator is assigned grade g if its ratio value is greater than Boundary (g-1) and less than or equal to Boundary (g).   Thus, a ratio of .45 for FEM-A is graded 1, and a ratio of 1.2 for FEM-C is graded 3.

It can be shown that the loss of information involved in grading continuous data into five categories, with boundaries specified, is slight (Ramsay, 1973). The gain, in this case, is the straightforward applicability of the latent trait model described previously with all its attendent advantages.   Because the functional relationship of the ratio measurements to skeletal age is unknown, no alternative solution is immediately obvious.

TABLE   XXII

Category Boundaries
Used to Convert
the Ratio Measurements
into Graded Variables

	Boundaries			
	1	2	3	4
FEM-A	0.5	0.6	0.7	0.8
FEM-B	2.0	2.25	2.5	2.75
FEM-C	1.0	1.1	1.2	1.3
TIB-A	0.6	0.7	0.8	0.9
TIB-B	2.5	2.7	2.9	3.1
FIB-A	0.3	0.5	0.7	0.9

FITTING THE MODEL: RESULTS

The first step in fitting the latent trait model
to these data is the estimation of the indicator
parameters. The original data for the analysis were
graded data for the thirty-four indicators for the
3997 radiographs of males and the 3800 radiographs of
females described in Chapter III. The analyses of the
male and female data were performed separately, using
the computer program LOGOG (Kolakowski and Bock, 1973).

The resultant threshold (T) and discriminability
(d) parameters for the males are given in Table XXIII
and for the females in Table XXIV. Many of the interesting features of the parameter values will be dis-
cussed at length in Chapter VII, but a few points will
be noted here.

Indicators are most usefully recorded at ages near
their threshold ages, because in that region they yield
the greatest amount of information about maturity.
Furthermore, in the vicinity of a threshold value, an
indicator of high discriminability yields more information than one of lower discriminability. Among this
set of indicators, it should be noted that indicators
applicable at early ages, that is, with thresholds
below two years, show considerably higher discriminability values than indicators with thresholds at later
ages (FEM-A-E, TIB-A, TIB-C, and TIB-D make up the
early group). The high discriminability of these
indicators means that maturity can be estimated with
greater precision at early ages than later, when only
indicators of lower discriminability are available.
Nevertheless, the wide distribution of the threshold
values across the entire age range means that satisfactory maturity estimates should be possible at
all ages.

The somewhat anomalous threshold value for TIB-D
for boys, -0.6 years, results from the fact that, in
this sample, more than 50 percent of the boys are
already in grade 2 at the age of three months. Thus
the threshold value is an extrapolation from the extant

TABLE   XXIII

Parameters for the 34 Knee Indicators for Boys

Indicator	T_1	T_2	T_3	T_4	d
FEM–A	0.4927	1.3556	2.3016	3.2535	3.3850
FEM–B	1.3059	1.8793	2.4970	3.2306	3.3085
FEM–C	1.5012	1.8902	2.3689	2.9495	3.4007
FEM–D	0.3887	1.0153			8.1123
FEM–E	0.7425				2.9541
FEM–F	10.2670				0.6603
FEM–G	10.5215				0.7965
FEM–H	3.2573	7.0421			0.9974
FEM–J	9.3877				1.0495
FEM–K	11.6273	14.4242			1.2656
FEM–L	15.8842	17.4685			1.1802
FEM–M	14.8926	16.7409			1.3680
TIB–A	0.8021	2.3873	3.9525	5.3198	2.0906
TIB–B	5.0022	6.3704	8.2832	10.4988	1.0954
TIB–C	0.2593				5.7874
TIB–D	-0.5998				3.8376
TIB–E	10.5891				0.6324
TIB–F	6.6701				0.8272
TIB–G	8.8921				0.6968
TIB–H	12.4275				0.8747
TIB–J	12.4788				0.8136
TIB–K	13.7778				0.8246
TIB–L	5.8374				0.6711
TIB–M	6.9485				0.9780
TIB–N	13.7184				1.1528
TIB–P	14.3476				1.6923
TIB–Q	15.5487	16.8720			1.5435
TIB–R	15.4091	17.0061			1.5006
FIB–A	4.0168	5.1537	7.1053	10.3038	1.5329
FIB–B	4.8066				1.0331
FIB–C	3.9216	5.2099			1.6766
FIB–D	9.1037				0.5381
FIB–E	10.7483				1.0688
FIB–F	15.4750	16.9406	17.4944		1.4297

T_{1-4} = the thresholds;   d = discriminability.

TABLE   XXIV

Parameters for the 34 Knee Indicators for Girls

Indicator	T_1	T_2	T_3	T_4	d
FEM-A	0.4262	0.9984	1.7310	2.2797	5.2967
FEM-B	1.0527	1.3923	1.8824	2.3218	5.1501
FEM-C	1.0906	1.3853	1.6877	2.1105	4.0893
FEM-D	0.1760	0.7070			8.8509
FEM-E	0.3983				6.1887
FEM-F	7.7940				0.8969
FEM-G	9.1371				0.8435
FEM-H	2.3473	5.2808			1.0921
FEM-J	6.8544				1.3028
FEM-K	10.1851	13.6033			1.4524
FEM-L	14.1031	16.1175			1.4539
FEM-M	12.7177	15.3927			1.1920
TIB-A	0.5465	1.7483	2.9375	4.0092	2.3086
TIB-B	3.8412	4.8152	6.3514	8.3020	1.1638
TIB-C	0.2626				7.9769
TIB-D	0.2045				5.9186
TIB-E	10.6483				0.4269
TIB-F	6.0547				0.5827
TIB-G	6.4372				0.7277
TIB-H	11.5395				0.5995
TIB-J	11.6580				0.6234
TIB-K	12.1090				0.5323
TIB-L	4.5134				0.7345
TIB-M	5.3444				1.3322
TIB-N	11.3358				1.3783
TIB-P	12.7237				1.2275
TIB-Q	14.4654	15.5538			1.5017
TIB-R	14.4377	15.9258			1.3684
FIB-A	3.2539	4.1607	5.9869	8.7435	1.6149
FIB-B	3.4131				1.4950
FIB-C	2.9391	3.9057			1.8004
FIB-D	7.4448				0.6870
FIB-E	9.9732				0.9830
FIB-F	14.3938	15.4729	16.1145		1.3718

T_{1-4} = the thresholds;   d = discriminability.

data, and cannot be estimated as precisely as the thresholds for the other indicators.   TIB-D does, however,
remain a useful indicator.

Before discussing the goodness-of-fit statistics
and the information curves for the total skeletal age
estimation system, it is useful to examine the rela-
tionships among the data, the fitted curve, and information for an individual indicator.   Figure 73 shows
the fitted logistic function and data, in hanging
histogram form, for **FIB-E** in boys, in addition to the
square root of the indicator information curve.   **FIB-E**
is a binary indicator with a threshold value of
10.75 years for males; thus the fitted curve crosses
the 50 percent point at age 10.75 years.   It is clear

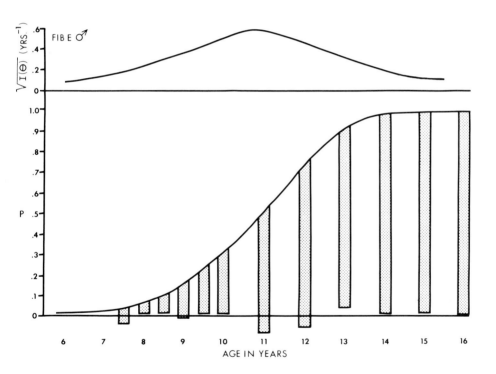

Figure 73. Hanging histogram of fitted logistic function
to the observed proportion of boys mature for **FIB-E** at
various ages and the associated information curve for
this indicator.

from Figure 73 that the fitted curve closely approximates the observed proportions (the shaded bars hanging
from the curve). At the top of Figure 73 is the ind-
cator information curve, which reflects the amount of
information from this indicator at various chronological
ages. The peak of the information curve is at the
threshold, 10.75 years, and the curve is rather flat,
reflecting the modest discriminability of this indicator (d = 1.07).

Figure 74 gives the corresponding picture for the
girls, which shows two major differences from the

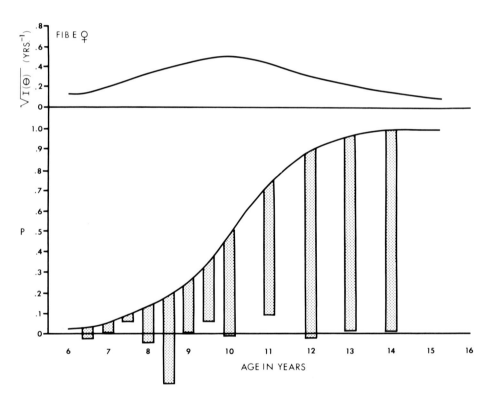

Figure 74. Hanging histogram of fitted logistic
function to the observed proportion of girls mature
for FIB-E at various ages and the associated information curve for this indicator.

results for the boys. The threshold for the girls is
9.98 years, almost a year earlier than that for the
boys, and the fit of the logistic to the data is less
good, especially at 8.5 and 11 years, where there are
deviations of the order of 20 percent and 10 percent
respectively. However, the data as a whole indicate
that the observed proportions at 8.5 and 11 years are
relatively deviant, and probably are due to sampling
peculiarities or measurement error. While the fit of
the model to these data is, therefore, not as good as
it is for the boys, the fit appears quite satisfactory
if the two deviant proportions are discounted.

The fitted curves and information functions for
indicator FEM-K for boys are shown in Figure 75, and
for girls in Figure 76. The observed prevalence data
are omitted from these more complicated figures for
purposes of clarity. Indicator FEM-K has three grades;
consequently, it has two threshold values, and thus the
information curves for this indicator have two peaks,
one at each threshold. For boys, the thresholds (and
regions of greatest information) are at 11.63 and
14.42 years, and for girls they are at 10.19 and
13.60 years. Again, the thresholds are about a year
earlier for girls than for boys.

As represented in these figures, there are information curves for each indicator, reflecting the amount
of information available from that indicator at a given
skeletal age. The sum of all of these indicator information curves for each sex are the total system information curves represented in Figure 77. Technical
details about the information function $I(\theta)$ and its
computation are given in Samejima (1969). This is
information in the Fisherian sense: the inverse of the
error variance at θ, the estimated skeletal age. Thus,
the square root of the information function, which is
shown in Figure 77, is the inverse of the standard error
of estimate of θ.

There are several interesting features of the
information curves in Figure 77. The information available from these thirty-four maturity indicators is

extremely similar for boys and girls at almost all
levels of SA.   Information is quite high at early
skeletal ages, say before the age of 2 years.   This
occurs because, as mentioned earlier, all the indicators applicable during these years are of high discriminability.   At a skeletal age of one year, the
information is nearly the same for both males and
females: the square root of I (θ) is about 5, so the
standard error of estimate of skeletal ages of one year
is about one fifth, or 0.2 years.   For both sexes,
I (θ) drops until a skeletal age of about 5 years, and
remains at about 1.5 thereafter; this is equivalent to

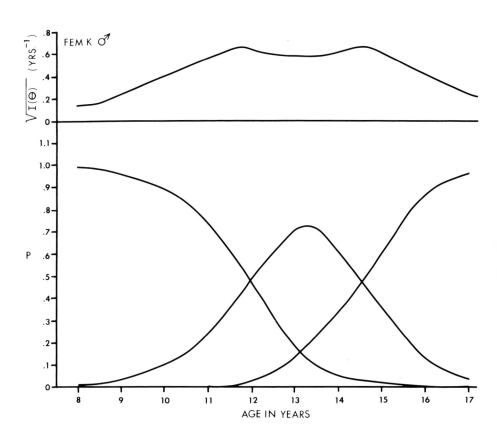

Figure 75.   Fitted logistic functions **FEM-K** in boys at
various ages and the associated information curve for
this indicator.

a standard error of about 0.66 years. The fluctuations
in the level of information are due to the passing of
threshold values (peaks of information) for various
indicators. While this is not strictly an indication
of goodness-of-fit of the model, it is clear from
Figure 77 that a good deal of information about skeletal
maturity is available from the thirty-four indicators
of the system. If more precision is required for a
particular range of skeletal age, further indicators
should be chosen that will have their thresholds in
that skeletal age range; their usefulness may be
examined by comparing the information curve for the
expanded system with the curves in Figure 77.

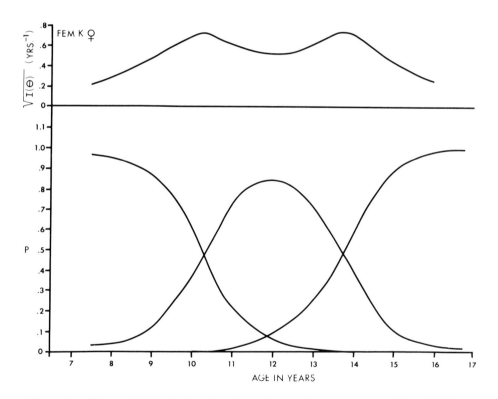

Figure 76. Fitted logistic functions **FEM-K** in girls at
various ages and the associated information curve for
this indicator.

The information curves show that the **RWT** method
for skeletal age assessment is precise enough to be
useful; but what about the goodness-of-fit statistics
for the model? The individual indicator and total
system Chi-square values (as described earlier, p. 190)
are listed in Table **XXV**. To give meaning to these
statistics, it will be useful to examine the Chi-square
values for **FIB-E**, the goodness-of-fit of which is
displayed graphically in Figures 73 and 74 for boys and
girls. The Chi-square value for **FIB-E** for boys is
27.85 (29 d.f.), which is nonsignificant, meaning that
no significant departure from the fitted model is
indicated. This conclusion agrees well with the
obvious good fit displayed in Figure 73. The Chi-
square for **FIB-E** for girls, on the other hand, is
42.22 (29 d.f.), which is significant (p < .05). This
indication of departure from fit is, of course, caused
by the deviations of the data from the fitted curve at
8.5 and 11 years. Thus, while the goodness-of-fit
Chi-square indicates a significant departure from fit,

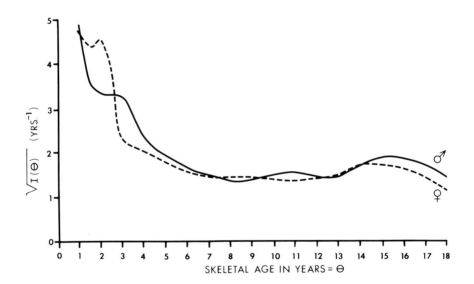

Figure 77. The total system information curves for the
RWT method at all ages for both sexes.

TABLE XXV

χ^2 Tests of Goodness-of-Fit for the
Logistic Model for the 34 Knee Indicators

Indicator	d.f.	Boys	Girls
FEM-A	119	195.97	148.58
FEM-B	119	175.77	110.12
FEM-C	119	133.05	125.46
FEM-D	59	97.17	55.61
FEM-E	29	38.29	47.65
FEM-F	29	140.04	57.74
FEM-G	29	58.73	60.53
FEM-H	59	192.95	238.56
FEM-J	29	34.93	91.89
FEM-K	59	62.84	42.68
FEM-L	59	60.55	55.96
FEM-M	59	52.67	53.31
TIB-A	119	136.68	159.87
TIB-B	119	461.19	462.54
TIB-C	29	31.19	41.54
TIB-D	29	75.37	24.26
TIB-E	29	103.95	108.00
TIB-F	29	215.47	267.71
TIB-G	29	35.75	55.40
TIB-H	29	21.15	145.92
TIB-J	29	56.07	143.24
TIB-K	29	71.78	133.89
TIB-L	29	123.92	129.50
TIB-M	29	50.59	30.49
TIB-N	29	33.30	115.16
TIB-P	29	23.19	40.35
TIB-Q	59	55.88	44.69
TIB-R	59	40.17	57.62
FIB-A	119	203.93	238.07
FIB-B	29	63.89	33.69
FIB-C	59	126.43	112.71
FIB-D	29	86.30	66.25
FIB-E	29	27.85	42.22
FIB-F	89	69.21	64.47
Total	1824	3358.87	3605.69

d.f. = degrees of freedom.

Figure 74 clearly shows that, except for two peculiar
proportions, the logistic fit does capture the essence
of the data.

The indicator Chi-squares, as a group, follow this
pattern: some show significant departures from fit, but
many do not. Those that show significant departures
from fit may be largely attributed to unusual proportions, such as that at age 8.5 for FIB-E for girls.
The total system Chi-square shows a significant departure from fit. But the total system information curves
have already shown that the system yields an adequate
amount of useful information about skeletal maturity.
So, while some indicators are clearly better than
others (both in the sense of yielding more information,
as shown by their higher discriminability, and in the
sense of fitting the logistic model better), all indicators may usefully continue to be included in the
estimation of skeletal maturity. The practical procedures for estimating skeletal maturity with these
indicators will be described in the next chapter.

CHAPTER VI

PROCEDURES FOR APPLYING THE RWT METHOD

Use of the RWT method to assign a skeletal age to a knee radiograph is very simple compared with the complex procedures involved in developing this method. Nevertheless, care is necessary so that indicator grades will be assigned with little error. The first need is that the radiographs be anteroposterior views of the left knee preferably taken at a tube-film distance of 91.4 cm (36 inches). The knee should be extended and the central ray directed at right angles to the long axes of the femur and tibia at the level of the joint.

PREPARATION AND TRAINING

The person who will do the assessing, called the "assessor" in the remainder of this chapter, should begin by reading the whole of this volume. He should acquire a suitable ruler (p. 71) and arrange the necessary computer services. The latter will involve using the small program for age estimation provided as Appendix II and organizing access to a central computer or use of a small desk computer with a memory of at least 40K. He will also need a stock of recording forms similar to the example in Table XXVI.

The assessor should begin his training by assessing a set of the test radiographs that are available (see p. 72). Of course, these should be assessed blind without reference to the listing of grades assigned by others, who are experienced with this method. After

all the test radiographs have been assessed, the
assessor should compare his ratings with those provided.

The assessments should be made in a dimly lit room.
The less light the better for viewing radiographs but,
if the room is too dark, the assessor will be unable to
read the parts of this book to which he will need to
refer continuously. The radiograph should be placed on

TABLE XXVI

Recording Sheet for RWT Skeletal Age

Name _____ C.A._____ Sex_____

Date of x-ray_____ Assessor_____

FEM-A:(MW) ____ FEM-J: ____ TIB-F:____ FIB-A:(MW)____

  " :(EW) ____ FEM-K: ____ TIB-G:____   " :(EW)____

FEM-B:(EH) ____ FEM-L: ____ TIB-H:____ FIB-B: ____

FEM-C:(WLC)____ FEM-M: ____ TIB-J:____ FIB-C: ____

  " :(HLC)____ TIB-A:(MW)____ TIB-K:____ FIB-D: ____

FEM-D: ____   " :(EW)____ TIB-L:____ FIB-E: ____

FEM-E: ____ TIB-B:(EH)____ TIB-M:____ FIB-F: ____

FEM-F: ____ TIB-C: ____ TIB-N:____

FEM-G: ____ TIB-D: ____ TIB-P:____

FEM-H: ____ TIB-E: ____ TIB-Q:____

                               TIB-R:____

Estimated S.A._____ years   s.e._____ years

a conveniently inclined transilluminated table with the proximal end of the radiograph away from the assessor and the lateral side of the knee to his left.   A plastic sheet containing the curves and lines shown in Figure 14 should be taken from the pocket at the back of this book.

The assessor should grade the indicators appropriate for the age and sex of the child (Tables XXIII and XXIV), recording his findings on the special recording form. When all the necessary indicators have been graded, the recorded data should be transferred to the computer. The output from the computer will be an estimate of the skeletal age and the standard error of this estimate. If the skeletal age is markedly divergent from the chronological age, the assessor should proceed to rate any additional indicators that are appropriate for the skeletal age level of the child. These additional data, together with those recorded earlier, should be transferred to the computer to obtain a revised and more accurate estimate of skeletal age.

INTERPRETATION

This subject will not be considered in full because satisfactory reviews are available concerning the effects of illness, socioeconomic factors, nutrition, climate and other factors on the rates of skeletal maturation (Tanner, 1962; Roche, 1965; Acheson, 1966; Roche et al., 1975).

The person interpreting the assessment should, at first, compare the estimated skeletal age with chronological age--this will help to indicate whether the child is advanced or retarded assuming that the mean skeletal maturity levels of the group (ethnic, socioeconomic, etc.) to which the child belongs match those of the standardizing sample of Southwestern Ohio children of middle socioeconomic status against which the RWT method was scaled. Of course, skeletal maturity levels vary within a group of normal children.

TABLE   XXVII

Indicators To Be Observed
at Particular Ages

BOYS

1 mo.–9 mos.	FEM	A,D,E
	TIB	A,C,D
1–1½ years	FEM	A,B,C,D,E,H
	TIB	A,C,D,F,L
	FIB	B,C
2 years	FEM	A,B,C,D,E,H
	TIB	A,D,F,L
	FIB	B,C
2½ years	FEM	A,B,C,E,H
	TIB	A,F,G,L,M
	FIB	B,C
3 years	FEM	A,B,C,H
	TIB	A,F,G,L,M
	FIB	B,C
3½–4 years	FEM	A,B,C,H
	TIB	A,F,G,L,M
	FIB	A,B,C,D
4½ years	FEM	A,B,C,H
	TIB	A,B,F,G,L,M
	FIB	A,B,C,D
5 years	FEM	A,B,C,H,J
	TIB	A,B,E,F,G,L,M
	FIB	A,B,C,D
5½ years	FEM	A,B,C,F,G,H,J
	TIB	A,B,E,F,G,L,M
	FIB	A,B,C,D
6 years	FEM	A,B,F,G,H,J
	TIB	A,B,E,F,G,L,M
	FIB	A,B,C,D
6½ years	FEM	A,F,G,H,J
	TIB	A,B,E,F,G,L,M
	FIB	A,B,C,D

(cont.)

TABLE XXVII (cont.)

7-7½ years	FEM	F, G, H, J
	TIB	A, B, E, F, G, H, J, L, M
	FIB	A, B, C, D, E
8-8½ years	FEM	F, G, H, J, K
	TIB	A, B, E, F, G, H, J, L, M
	FIB	A, B, C, D, E
9 years	FEM	F, G, H, J, K
	TIB	A, B, E, F, G, H, J, K, L, M
	FIB	A, B, C, D, E
9½ years	FEM	F, G, H, J, K
	TIB	A, B, E, F, G, H, J, K, L, M
	FIB	A, D, E
10 years	FEM	F, G, H, J, K
	TIB	A, B, E, F, G, H, J, K, L, M, N
	FIB	A, D, E
11 years	FEM	F, G, H, J, K, L, M
	TIB	B, E, F, G, H, J, K, M, N, R
	FIB	A, D, E, F
12 years	FEM	F, G, J, K, L, M
	TIB	B, E, F, G, H, J, K, M, N, P, Q, R
	FIB	A, D, E, F
13-14 years	FEM	F, G, J, K, L, M
	TIB	E, F, G, H, J, K, N, P, Q, R
	FIB	A, D, E, F
15 years	FEM	F, J, K, L, M
	TIB	E, H, J, K, N, P, Q, R
	FIB	A, D, E, F
16 years	FEM	F, J, K, L, M
	TIB	E, H, J, K, N, P, Q, R
	FIB	A, E, F
17 years	FEM	F, J, K, L, M
	TIB	E, H, J, K, N, P, Q, R
	FIB	F
18 years	FEM	F, L, M
	TIB	E, H, J, K, Q, R
	FIB	F

TABLE   XXVIII

Indicators To Be Observed
at Particular Ages

GIRLS

| 1 month | FEM | A,D,E |
| | TIB | A,C,D |

3-6 months	FEM	A,D,E
	TIB	A,C,D
	FIB	B

9 months	FEM	A,B,C,D,E,H
	TIB	A,C,D,L
	FIB	B

1 year	FEM	A,B,C,D,E,H
	TIB	A,C,D,F,L
	FIB	B,C

1½ years	FEM	A,B,C,D,E,H
	TIB	A,C,F,G,L
	FIB	B,C

2 years	FEM	A,B,C,D,E,H
	TIB	A,F,G,L
	FIB	B,C,D

2½ years	FEM	A,B,C,H
	TIB	A,F,G,L,M
	FIB	B,C,D

3 years	FEM	A,B,C,F,H
	TIB	A,E,F,G,L,M
	FIB	A,B,C,D

3½ years	FEM	A,B,C,F,H
	TIB	A,B,E,F,G,L,M
	FIB	A,B,C,D

(cont.)

TABLE XXVIII (cont.)

4 years	FEM	A, B, F, G, H
	TIB	A, B, E, F, G, L, M
	FIB	A, B, C, D
4½-5½ years	FEM	A, B, F, G, H, J
	TIB	A, B, E, F, G, L, M
	FIB	A, B, C, D
6-6½ years	FEM	F, G, H, J
	TIB	A, B, E, F, G, K, L, M
	FIB	A, B, C, D, E
7 years	FEM	F, G, H, J
	TIB	A, B, E, F, G, H, J, K, L, M
	FIB	A, B, C, D, E
7½-8 years	FEM	F, G, H, J, K
	TIB	A, B, E, F, G, H, J, K, L, M
	FIB	A, D, E
8½ years	FEM	F, G, H, J, K
	TIB	A, B, E, F, G, H, J, K, L, M, N
	FIB	A, D, E
9 years	FEM	F, G, H, J, K, M
	TIB	A, B, E, F, G, H, J, K, L, M, N
	FIB	A, D, E
9½ years	FEM	F, G, H, J, K, M
	TIB	A, B, E, F, G, H, J, K, N, P
	FIB	A, D, E
10 years	FEM	F, G, H, J, K, M
	TIB	A, B, E, F, G, H, J, K, N, P
	FIB	A, D, E, F
11 years	FEM	F, G, H, J, K, L, M
	TIB	B, E, F, G, H, J, K, N, P, Q, R
	FIB	A, D, E, F

(continued)

TABLE XXVIII (cont.)

12 years   FEM   F, G, K, L, M
                TIB   B, E, F, G, H, J, K, N, P, Q, R
                FIB   A, D, E, F

13 years   FEM   F, G, K, L, M
                TIB   E, F, H, J, K, N, P, Q, R
                FIB   A, D, E, F

14 years   FEM   G, K, L, M
                TIB   E, F, H, J, K, N, P, Q, R
                FIB   A, D, E, F

15 years   FEM   G, K, L, M
                TIB   E, F, H, J, K, N, P, Q, R
                FIB   F

16 years   FEM   K, L, M
                TIB   E, F, H, J, K, N, P, Q, R
                FIB   F

17 years   FEM   L, M
                TIB   E, H, J, K, P, Q, R
                FIB   F

18 years   FEM   L, M
                TIB   E, H, J, K, Q, R
                FIB   F

Usually, in data distributed in an approximately normal
fashion, as is the case with skeletal age except near
the end of the scale, the range from -2 s.d. to +2 s.d.
is considered "normal." The data needed to calculate
the limits of normal are given in Table XXVI. Only
children outside this range should be labelled "accelerated" or "retarded" and should be investigated.
Despite the presence of skewness near the ends of the
skeletal maturity scale, it is reasonable to apply the
same criterion of the normal range (± 2 s.d.) at all
chronological ages. If assessments of serial radiographs are being interpreted, it is necessary to
consider the change in level of a child across age.
A child may shift from -1.5 s.d. to +1.5 s.d. while
remaining in the normal range. Such a change may be
important. Consequently, it should be noted and its
cause sought.

It is necessary for the assessor to recall that
acceleration or retardation of skeletal maturation can
be caused by a wide variety of unrelated factors.
view is equally important: a normal level of skeletal
maturity means little more than that--few pathological
conditions can be excluded by such a finding.

Having evaluated whether the estimated skeletal
age is outside the normal range, the assessor should
direct his attention to the standard error of the estimate for the individual radiograph. This shows the
level of accuracy of the estimate. It is appropriate
to allow ± 1.5 s.e. of the estimate of skeletal age as
the range (95 percent confidence limits) within which
the actual, but generally unknown, skeletal age will lie.

These principles can be illustrated by examples.
If an assessment were made of a boy aged 10 years, the
estimate of his RWT skeletal age might be 10.4 years
with a standard error of 0.2 years. The low standard
error shows the estimate is relatively accurate and
that his actual skeletal age is between 10.1 and
10.7 years (95 percent confidence limits). It can be
concluded that his skeletal maturity level is within
the normal range. If a radiograph of a girl aged 2 years

were assessed, the estimated skeletal age might be
1.5 years with a standard error of the estimate of
0.3 years. The actual skeletal age of this girl will
be in the range of 1.05 to 1.95 years. At 2.0 years
(CA), the normal range of skeletal age for girls is
1.18 to 2.94 years (Table XXVI). Consequently, this
girl would tend to be slightly retarded but it is
highly likely that her actual skeletal age is within
the normal range.

CHAPTER VII

SOME FINDINGS WITH THE RWT METHOD

The RWT method allowed skeletal age assessments to be made for almost all the participants in the Fels Longitudinal Study except towards the ends of the distribution of chronological ages when increasing proportions in each age group could not be assessed (Table XXIX). Even at the ends of the distribution, a higher proportion of these children and youths could be assessed with the RWT method than with the current alternatives (Greulich and Pyle, 1959; Tanner et al., 1962, 1972, 1975; Pyle and Hoerr, 1969).

It is most important that the method allow a high proportion to be assessed. It is, however, equally important that each assessment be based on data capable of yielding an accurate skeletal age for the individual. Put another way, the estimates must have standard errors known to be small. In theory, the methods that are alternatives to the RWT method that is described in this book could be applied to every child at all ages; their restriction to children in whom sufficient information is available is dependent on the subjective judgment of the assessor. With the RWT method this restriction is included in the computer program.

LEVELS AND DISTRIBUTIONS

The RWT method was scaled so that the mean of the derived skeletal ages would be equal to the mean chronological age for the group. Consequently, it is, of course, not surprising that the mean skeletal and chronological ages for the participants in the Fels

Longitudinal Study are related in a linear fashion
(Figure 78). The only appreciable divergence between
the mean chronological and skeletal ages occurs at older
ages (18 years, boys; 17 and 18 years, girls) when the
mean skeletal ages are less than the mean chronological
ages by 0.4 to 1.1 years (Table XXX). These comparatively large differences occur because not all the
radiographs could be assessed at these ages. Some were
completely mature, making it impossible to assign a

Table XXIX

The Proportion of Participants
in the Fels Longitudinal Study
for Whom Skeletal Age
Assessments Could Be Made

Chronological age (years)	Boys	Girls
0.1	0.49	0.60
0.3	0.92	0.94
0.5	0.98	0.99
0.8	----	----
1.0	----	0.99
1.5	----	----
12.0	----	0.99
13.0	----	0.96
14.0	----	0.95
15.0	----	0.93
16.0	0.92	0.86
17.0	0.81	0.55
18.0	0.59	0.51

---- = all participants
could be assessed.

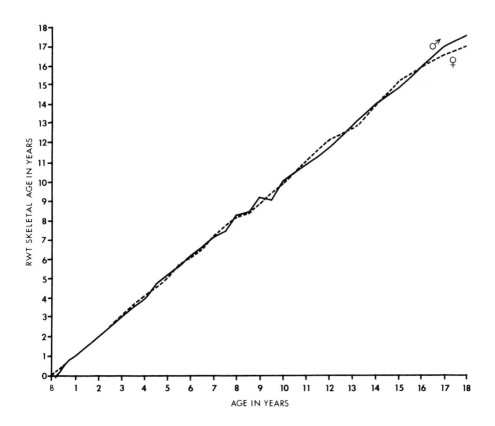

Figure 78.   Mean RWT skeletal ages within chronological age groups for children in the Fels Longitudinal Study.

TABLE   XXX

Means and Standard Deviations of Skeletal Age
in the Fels Longitudinal Study

Chronological Age (years)	Boys			Girls		
	N	Mean	s.d.	N	Mean	s.d.
.1	55	-0.05	0.24	75	0.12	0.11
.3	80	0.16	0.25	94	0.32	0.16
.5	125	0.54	0.28	140	0.54	0.19
.8	83	0.80	0.25	99	0.84	0.25
1.0	164	1.06	0.31	140	1.04	0.26
1.5	108	1.50	0.42	114	1.52	0.36
2.0	157	2.08	0.41	136	2.05	0.47
2.5	105	2.52	0.46	108	2.55	0.47
3.0	149	3.00	0.49	133	3.12	0.72
3.5	98	3.55	0.59	100	3.67	0.79
4.0	151	3.95	0.63	132	4.17	0.92
4.5	100	4.73	0.79	89	4.63	0.89
5.0	140	5.24	0.96	123	5.08	0.98
5.5	90	5.72	0.98	74	5.76	0.91
6.0	213	6.14	0.98	195	6.08	0.95
6.5	117	6.68	0.96	100	6.51	1.01
7.0	201	7.15	0.95	204	7.13	0.91
7.5	113	7.45	0.93	96	7.72	0.98
8.0	187	8.24	0.99	189	8.15	0.94
8.5	112	8.45	1.08	93	8.38	1.18
9.0	182	9.15	1.08	175	8.88	1.09
9.5	47	9.09	1.47	80	9.35	1.03
10.0	175	9.98	.99	166	9.91	1.14
11.0	149	10.81	1.05	137	11.02	1.16
12.0	135	11.70	1.05	133	12.11	1.02
13.0	132	13.02	1.03	114	12.79	0.83
14.0	124	13.95	1.12	112	13.88	1.10
15.0	102	14.80	1.13	99	15.10	1.30
16.0	97	15.87	1.03	88	15.84	1.13
17.0	79	16.86	1.13	41	16.42	0.81
18.0	54	17.49	.88	26	16.88	0.60

skeletal age. Consequently, the group of radiographs
that was assessed at older ages contained a dispropor-
tionate number of those that were relatively less mature.

The distributions of skeletal age are skewed
significantly within some chronological age groups in
each sex. The direction of this skewness varies,
especially in the boys, being more often to the right
than the left. As would be expected from the truncated
nature of the skeletal maturity scale, skewness to the
right is relatively common at young ages; at older ages
skewness to the left is more common. The extent of
the skewness is not sufficient to make it necessary
that percentiles be used to describe the distributions
of skeletal ages within chronological age groups.

Expectedly, the standard deviations increase in
each sex until about 4.5 years, after which there is
no consistent trend except for a decrease in girls
after 15 years (Figure 79). This decrease occurs
because the skeletal maturity scale has an upper limit
that girls tend to reach at younger ages than do boys.
There are no appreciable sex differences in the variance
except from 2.5 through 4 years when it is greater in
the girls and at 17 and 18 years when the variance is
greater in the boys. The variance does not increase at
puberty, which would be expected if, as the literature
indicates (Flory, 1936; Hewitt and Acheson, 1961a;
Roche et al., in press), skeletal maturation is accelerated at puberty with this acceleration occurring at
different chronological ages among individuals.

The coefficient of variation [100(s.d.)/mean]
decreases rapidly to 2 years (with some irregularity
in the girls) and later more slowly in an almost linear
fashion. There is no appreciable sex difference in
these coefficients (Figure 80). Values prior to
0.75 years were omitted from the figure.

As with all other assessment methods, the variance
of RWT skeletal age has two components: the true variance of skeletal maturity level which reflects actual
variations among individuals in skeletal maturity
levels and errors due to the limited ability of

TABLE   XXXI

Percentiles of Standard Errors for RWT Skeletal Age
in the Fels Longitudinal Study

Chronological	Boys			Girls		
Age (years)	10	50	90	10	50	90
.1	.21	.31	.42	.13	.15	.18
.3	.19	.21	.42	.13	.15	.16
.5	.19	.21	.25	.13	.15	.18
.8	.19	.21	.23	.16	.18	.23
1.0	.20	.23	.29	.16	.20	.30
1.5	.21	.26	.32	.19	.21	.42
2.0	.26	.27	.33	.20	.32	.43
2.5	.27	.28	.32	.21	.35	.46
3.0	.27	.30	.38	.25	.42	.49
3.5	.29	.35	.48	.32	.43	.53
4.0	.31	.43	.50	.38	.47	.57
4.5	.40	.49	.56	.42	.51	.59
5.0	.45	.52	.64	.44	.55	.69
5.5	.49	.55	.67	.51	.58	.67
6.0	.50	.60	.77	.54	.63	.92
6.5	.58	.72	.89	.59	.74	.88
7.0	.57	.66	.84	.60	.68	.82
7.5	.66	.79	.92	.73	.82	1.00
8.0	.64	.70	.82	.64	.69	.94
8.5	.72	.84	1.05	.69	.81	1.00
9.0	.65	.71	.89	.65	.69	.84
9.5	.75	1.02	1.38	.84	.96	1.33
10.0	.63	.70	.87	.66	.72	.96
11.0	.64	.69	.78	.67	.71	.88
12.0	.65	.71	.85	.64	.72	.93
13.0	.58	.69	.81	.59	.71	.91
14.0	.52	.65	.85	.54	.65	.87
15.0	.51	.61	.76	.52	.64	.89
16.0	.51	.58	.80	.54	.71	1.17
17.0	.52	.65	.88	.57	.81	1.18
18.0	.55	.75	1.02	.63	.80	1.24

The numbers in each age group are the same as
in Table XXVII.

errors until about 15 years.   In each sex, the standard
errors increase at later ages because few maturity
indicators are informative at these ages.   This
increase in the standard errors towards the end of the
skeletal maturity scale is more marked in the girls
than the boys, which reflects the well-known fact that
girls tend to reach adult levels of maturity at younger
ages than do boys.

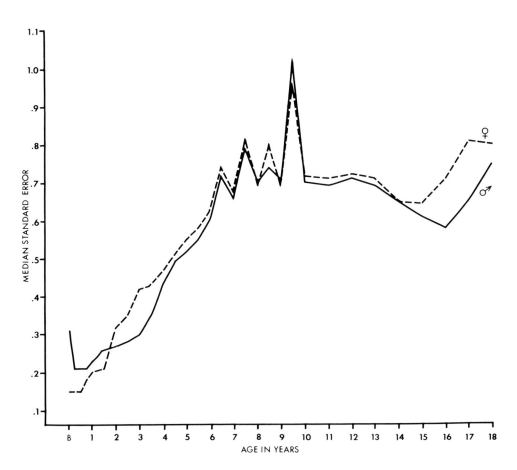

Figure 81.   Median standard errors of RWT skeletal ages
within chronological age groups for children in the
Fels Longitudinal Study.

If the standard errors are expressed relative to
the mean skeletal age thus:

$$\frac{100 \ (\text{median s.e.})}{\text{mean skeletal age}} ,$$

the irregularity across ages is reduced (Figure 82) and
the values decrease with chronological age at a
decelerating rate. Values prior to 0.5 years were
omitted from the figure.

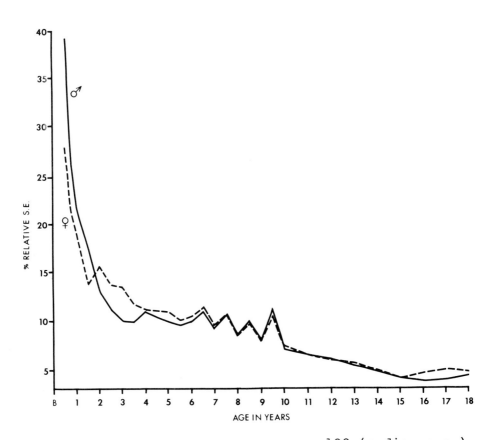

Figure 82. Relative standard errors $\dfrac{100 \ (\text{median s.e.})}{\text{mean skeletal age}}$
of RWT skeletal ages within chronological age groups
for children in the Fels Longitudinal Study.

The level of the median standard errors is about
0.7 years, except at ages before 6 years, when they
are smaller. The standard deviation of skeletal age
(which reflects the combined effects of actual variability and measurement error) is close to one year at
chronological ages of 6 years and older. Consequently,
a large proportion of the observed variation is due to
error. This is shown in Figure 83 as the proportion
s.e./s.d., which will be referred to as the relative
standard error. As can be seen from this figure, the
relative standard error is about 0.6 to 0.7 at all ages
in each sex, except at both ends of the age scale when
the proportions are considerably higher, particularly
for the girls. While attention has been directed to

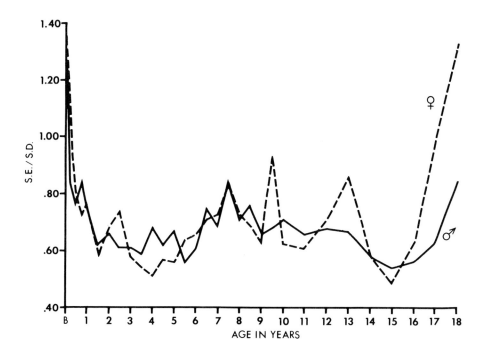

Figure 83. The proportion s.d./s.d. within chronological age groups for children in the Fels Longitudinal Study.

the large proportion of the variance that is due to
error, it should not be overlooked that these findings
lead to the additional and important conclusion that
the true variability of skeletal age within chronological age groups is considerably less than that
reported from studies based on methods that provide
only the total variability (true variability plus error).

SEX DIFFERENCES

    As described earlier (Chapter V), the findings for
each indicator provide prevalence data, grade by grade,
within chronological age groups for each sex. From
these data, ages were estimated within each sex at
which each grade was present in 50 percent of the group
(thresholds). The sex differences between these ages
(thresholds) provide information about sex differences
in the rates of development of individual maturity
indicators. In Figure 84, these sex differences are
plotted against the ages at which thresholds are
crossed (means of thresholds in males and females).
As expected, the thresholds are generally at younger
ages in girls than boys. The sex differences tend to
increase with the mean thresholds until about 6 years,
after which there is little systematic change. These
sex differences do not vary systematically among the
femur, tibia and fibula. The findings are of particular
interest because they are in such marked contrast to
findings for many anthropometric variables in which
there are no sex differences until about the age of
pubescence in girls (Tanner, 1962; Malina et al.,1973).
By contrast, there is a sex difference in the present
data from soon after birth and there is no increase
after 6 years. Figure 84 shows also that the sex differences in thresholds across indicator grades are
relatively uniform to 5 years but not at later ages.

    There are two very deviant values--these are the
two earliest values plotted for the tibia. The threshold for TIB-D (epiphyseal shape) that occurs in boys at
-0.6 years (Figure 108) was obtained by extrapolation.

The sex difference (-0.8 years) is unusually large for
an indicator with such an early threshold. Also it is
most unusual for a threshold for an indicator grade to
be reached earlier in boys than in girls. The uncer-
tainty of this particular estimate is clear from the
prevalence of indicator grades against age (Figure 108).
The calculated threshold for TIB-E (radio-opaque zone
due to lateral articular surface) also is earlier in
boys than girls (Figure 109) but the difference is very
small (-0.06 years).

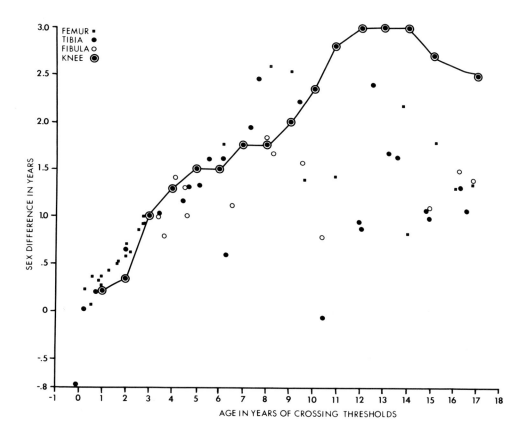

Figure 84. Differences between boys and girls in the
Fels Longitudinal Study in the ages at which thresholds
are crossed for each grade of every indicator. The
data for the "knee" are from Roche (1968).

The somewhat relevant data reported previously do
not refer to separate maturity indicators except ages
at onset of ossification and epiphyseo-diaphyseal
fusion. Ages at onset of ossification are reasonably
accurate for the fibular epiphysis only; the femoral
and tibial epiphyses begin to ossify before or near
birth making it very difficult to estimate accurately
the ages at which ossification begins. The thresholds
from the present study correspond closely to the mean
or median ages reported previously for the onset of
ossification in the fibular epiphysis in United States
children (Table XXXI).

The only reported data for epiphyseo-diaphyseal
fusion at the knee joint in United States children are
from Pyle et al. (1961) and Hansman (1962). The
thresholds from the present study are later than those
reported previously but some of the differences are
small (Table XXXII). These differences could be due in
part, to variations among investigators in their
criteria for the completion of epiphyseal fusion

TABLE XXXI

Modal Ages at Onset of Ossification
in the Proximal Fibular Epiphysis in
United States Children (years)

	Boys	Girls
Greulich and Pyle (1959)	3.9	2.9
Pyle et al. (1961)	3.8	3.0
Hansman (1962)	4.4	3.1
Garn et al. (1967)	3.5	2.6
RWT thresholds	3.9	2.9

although the written descriptions of the criteria are
closely similar. Diversity of criteria, however, is
unlikely to be responsible for the apparent differences
in the sequence of fusion across bones when the findings
of Hansman (1962) are compared with those from the present study. In Hansman's data, the order in each sex is
femur, tibia, fibula. In the present data, the order in
each sex is tibia followed by the femur and fibula,
which are tied. The data of Hansman indicate that the
sex differences in the timing of fusion at the knee
joint are about 2.0 years; these are slightly greater
than those found in the present study which is based on
a much larger group.

It is well known that the knee joint is more mature
in girls than boys at birth (Menees and Holly, 1932;
Kessler and Scott, 1950). Sex differences at later
ages have been reported by Roche (1968) who assessed
the male standards in one copy of the Pyle and Hoerr
atlas against the female standards in another copy.
The differences reported by Roche, expressed in male

TABLE XXXII

Modal Ages at Completion of Epiphyseo-Diaphyseal
Fusion in United States Youths (years)

	Pyle et al. (1961)	Hansman (1962)	RWT thresholds
Femur			
male	----	16.6	17.5
female	----	14.7	16.1
Tibia			
male	----	16.9	17.0
female	----	14.8	15.9
Fibula			
male	17.0	17.2	17.5
female	15.7	15.2	16.1

skeletal age years, are included in Figure 84 where
they are identified as "knee." These sex differences
for the knee as a whole are close to the general trend
for individual indicators in the present study except
after 11 years when the area differences are greater by
about 1.5 years. Perhaps, after 11 years, the sex
differences in level between the Pyle and Hoerr atlas
standards are too large, as has been shown for the
Greulich and Pyle hand-wrist atlas standards at ages
after 13 years (Roche et al., 1974 and in press).

The sex difference for each threshold of every
indicator grade has been considered also as a percentage of the conception corrected mean age, i.e., the
mean of the chronological ages for the crossing of the
threshold by males and females after adding 0.75 years
(approximate gestation period) to these ages. It
could be hypothesized that this age correction would
remove much of the systematic variation in the extent
of the sex differences between the thresholds crossed
early compared with those crossed late. In fact, this
did occur as can be seen in Figure 85 where these
percentages are plotted against the mean ages (males
and females) at which the thresholds are crossed.
The ages on the x axis are not conception-corrected.
TIB-D (epiphyseal shape) remains divergent. This
maturity indicator is so different in this respect
(-1.45 at -0.2 years) that it has been omitted from the
figure. As noted earlier, the threshold for TIB-D in
the boys was obtained by extrapolation. Consequently,
neither the value for the boys nor the sex differences
are as reliable as the corresponding estimates for
other maturity indicators.

Inspection of Figure 85 shows that the conception
corrected sex differences are about 20 percent until
9 years, after which the values decrease gradually
until they are about 7 percent at 14 years and over.
These sex differences are markedly variable even for
maturity indicators that cross thresholds at about the
same age. This variability is present at all ages
except at 14 years and over. The pattern of change
with age in this variability is not due to selective

sampling--all the appropriate indicators were rated in each radiograph. Sex differences in maturity levels obtained using the atlas method are made more difficult to interpret by the fact that, at early ages, the comparisons tend to be between all the girls and the accelerated boys and at older ages they are between the slowly maturing girls and all the boys.

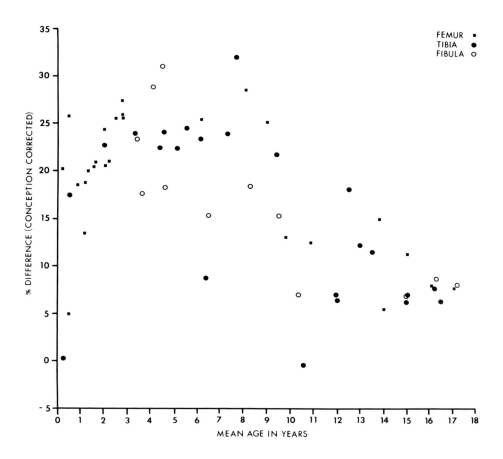

Figure 85. Sex differences in the ages at which thresholds are crossed for indicator grades expressed as the percentage of the conception-corrected mean age. These data are from children in the Fels Longitudinal Study. See text for details.

The data recorded during the present study allow
an analysis of possible sex differences in the sequence
of indicators for the bones of the knee joint. This
can be done simply by considering sex differences in
the order in which thresholds for indicator grades are
crossed. In Figure 86, the sequence in which the
thresholds for each indicator grade are crossed in boys
has been plotted against the corresponding sequence in
girls. If there were an exact match between the sexes,

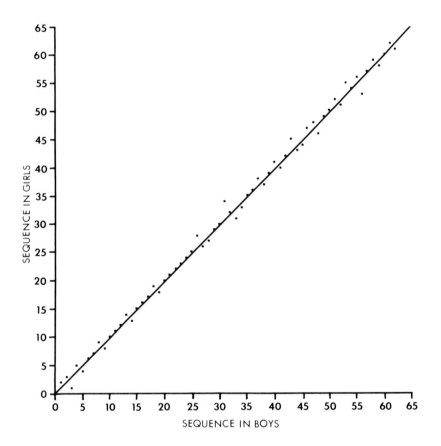

Figure 86. The sequence in which thresholds for
indicator grades were crossed in boys plotted against
the corresponding sequence in girls. These data are
from the Fels Longitudinal Study.

all these points would lie on the straight line included
in the figure. Clearly, the deviation from an exact
match is small--the largest divergence is three places
(for two indicators, TIB-F and FEM-L, Grade 2 and 3).
Such a close correspondence for the 62 grades considered
shows the sequence of maturation is the same in each sex.
This leads to the conclusion that Pyle and Hoerr (1969)
were justified in constructing a single series of standards for the maturation of the knee in both sexes.
It should be recalled, however, that the presence of
the adductor tubercle was omitted from the list of
indicators used in the RWT method because it became
universal only in the boys, not the girls.

REPLICABILITY

The replicability (repeatability) of RWT assessments was tested by using 80 radiographs (10 of each
sex at ages 2, 6, 10 and 14 years). Every radiograph
was assessed twice by each of two observers acting
independently, thus providing data for the calculation
of inter- and intra-observer differences. The sets of
indicator grades assigned to the same radiograph varied,
as would be expected, because the categories used are
mostly artificial divisions in biological continua.

A complete set of data was processed by the computer; all of the possible 80 skeletal ages were
estimated. Very near each end of the skeletal
maturity scale, there were few useful indicators and
some individuals were assigned many completely immature
or completely mature indicator grades in one or more of
the four assessments. Nevertheless, skeletal ages could
be assigned to all the radiographs. This is notable
because, at any age, but more commonly near each end
of the skeletal maturity scale, a very unusual pattern
of skeletal maturity grades within a radiograph may
make it impossible to estimate skeletal age accurately with the data available. No matter how large
the sample, there will always be unusual combinations

or patterns of indicator grades assigned to some radiographs. A priori, the number of unusual patterns must
be small; therefore, there will be insufficient information to allow accurate estimates of the skeletal ages
that should be assigned to such radiographs.

   Distribution statistics relating to the inter-
and intra-observer differences are given in Table XXXIII.
These show median differences ranging from 0.1 to
0.3 years approximately. These are lower than those
generally reported by others when using the atlas
method (Mainland, 1954; Demisch and Wartmann, 1956;
Gray and Lamons, 1959; Hansman and Maresh, 1961; Koski
et al., 1961; Moed et al., 1962; Acheson et al., 1963;
Johnston, 1963; Anderson et al., 1965; Anderson, 1967;
Andersen, 1968; Roche et al., 1970, 1974; Mazess and
Cameron, 1971; Sproul and Peritz, 1971).

   The next aspect of replicability considered is the
prevalence of differences between the grades assigned
to individual indicators (Table XXXIV). These differences do not exceed two grades--almost all of them were

TABLE   XXXIII

Percentiles of Inter- and Intra-Observer
Differences in Years from RWT Assessments
(All Ages Combined)

	N	Percentiles		
		10	50	90
Inter-observer	80	0.02	0.26	0.80
Intra-observer (A)	80	0.0	0.18	0.71
Intra-observer (B)	80	0.0	0.08	0.59

TABLE   XXXII

Percentage Prevalence of Differences between Grades of
Indicators Assigned to the Same Radiographs (N = 80)

Indicator	Inter-observer		Intra-observer A		Intra-observer B	
	1	2	1	2	1	2
FEM-A	3.7	0.0	5.0	0.0	1.2	0.0
FEM-B	5.0	0.0	5.0	0.0	2.5	0.0
FEM-C	8.7	5.0	8.7	2.5	8.7	0.0
FEM-D	0.0	0.0	0.0	0.0	0.0	0.0
FEM-E	1.3	0.0	0.0	0.0	1.3	0.0
FEM-F	3.7	0.0	2.6	0.0	1.2	0.0
FEM-G	9.9	0.0	13.7	0.0	6.8	0.0
FEM-H	17.7	0.0	10.3	0.0	5.0	0.0
FEM-J	6.3	0.0	1.2	0.0	3.7	0.0
FEM-K	10.0	0.0	5.0	0.0	5.0	0.0
FEM-L	2.5	0.0	3.7	0.0	0.0	0.0
FEM-M	5.2	0.0	2.6	0.0	2.5	0.0
TIB-A	2.5	0.0	2.5	0.0	1.2	0.0
TIB-B	5.0	0.0	8.7	0.0	7.5	1.2
TIB-C	0.0	0.0	0.0	0.0	0.0	0.0
TIB-D	0.0	0.0	0.0	0.0	0.0	0.0
TIB-E	10.0	0.0	5.0	0.0	3.7	0.0
TIB-F	0.0	0.0	5.0	0.0	1.2	0.0
TIB-G	6.3	0.0	5.1	0.0	3.8	0.0
TIB-H	5.0	0.0	6.3	0.0	0.0	0.0
TIB-J	8.7	0.0	5.0	0.0	6.3	0.0
TIB-K	12.5	0.0	3.8	0.0	3.7	0.0
TIB-L	11.4	0.0	8.6	0.0	2.9	0.0
TIB-M	4.4	0.0	7.2	0.0	1.5	0.0
TIB-N	2.6	0.0	2.6	0.0	1.3	0.0
TIB-P	2.5	0.0	2.5	0.0	0.0	0.0
TIB-Q	2.6	0.0	1.3	0.0	2.5	0.0
TIB-R	5.0	0.0	2.5	1.3	1.2	0.0
FIB-A	1.3	0.0	5.0	0.0	1.3	0.0
FIB-B	1.3	0.0	3.9	0.0	0.0	0.0
FIB-C	1.2	0.0	0.0	0.0	0.0	0.0
FIB-D	14.8	0.0	7.3	0.0	1.7	0.0
FIB-E	3.8	0.0	2.6	0.0	1.2	0.0
FIB-F	8.7	0.0	7.5	0.0	2.5	0.0

differences of one grade. There are many indicators
for which the prevalence of differences is low, and
some in which no differences are observed at all. The
indicators with the highest prevalence of differences
are FEM-C (ratio width lateral condyle/height lateral
condyle) and FEM-G (transverse trabeculae) but even in
these, the prevalence is not very high.

Next the percentage prevalence of differences was
considered within each bone for all indicators combined
and for the knee as a whole (Table XXXV).   The prevalence of differences is low but is slightly greater for
the femur than for either of the other bones or the
knee as a whole.

COMPARISONS WITH RATINGS BY OTHER METHODS

Attempts were made to assess skeletal age at
various chronological ages in radiographs of the same
group of children, using two methods for the knee (RWT
and Pyle and Hoerr, 1969) and two methods for the hand-
wrist (Greulich and Pyle, 1959; Tanner et al., 1972,
1975). At each end of the scale, a larger proportion

TABLE   XXXV

Percentage Prevalence of Differences between Grades of
Indicators Assigned to the Same Radiographs by Bone and
for the Whole Area (N=80)

Bone or area	Inter-observer		Intra-observer A		Intra-observer B	
	1	2	1	2	1	2
Femur	6.1	0.4	4.8	0.2	3.2	0
Tibia	4.9	0	4.1	0.1	2.3	0.1
Fibula	4.7	0	4.2	0	1.1	0
Knee	5.0	0.5	4.4	0.1	2.4	0.1

of the radiographs could be assessed with the RWT
method than with any of the other methods.

Table XXXVI provides the mean differences between
the knee skeletal ages assigned to these radiographs
using the RWT and Pyle and Hoerr methods.   The sample
at each age varies from 15 to 117.   The relative differences do not vary systematically from zero in the
boys except from 5 through 9 years when they are all
positive; this implies that the Pyle and Hoerr scale

TABLE   XXXVI

Mean Differences (Years) between RWT and
Pyle-Hoerr Skeletal Ages (Knee) for
Children in the Fels Longitudinal Study

Chronological age	Relative		Absolute	
	Boys	Girls	Boys	Girls
0.1	-0.12	0.04	0.20	0.10
0.3	-0.14	-0.01	0.22	0.10
0.5	-0.08	-0.05	0.20	0.11
0.8	-0.07	0.11	0.22	0.16
1.0	0.03	0.10	0.24	0.22
1.5	0.01	0.10	0.28	0.21
2.0	0.02	0.11	0.26	0.30
2.5	-0.11	0.10	0.32	0.25
3.0	-0.16	0.17	0.32	0.44
3.5	-0.23	0.25	0.43	0.42
4.0	-0.21	0.37	0.39	0.58
4.5	0.04	0.30	0.49	0.49
5.0	0.14	0.35	0.61	0.56
5.5	0.26	0.54	0.63	0.60
6.0	0.43	0.41	0.69	0.69
7.0	0.41	0.63	0.65	0.77
8.0	0.37	0.79	0.68	0.89
9.0	0.20	0.76	0.62	0.91
10.0	-0.01	0.71	0.59	1.00
11.0	-0.10	0.69	0.67	1.05
12.0	-0.41	0.59	0.81	0.87
13.0	-0.27	0.44	0.65	0.64
14.0	-0.69	0.57	0.93	0.72
15.0	-0.22	1.02	0.66	1.08
16.0	0.06	0.79	0.78	0.81

for boys is set too high for the Fels group during this
age range. An opposite tendency is present from 10
through 15 years when the Pyle and Hoerr scale is set
slightly too low for the Fels boys. In the girls, the
differences are positive at all ages and, in general,
increase as later chronological ages are considered.
The Pyle and Hoerr scale is set too high for these Fels
girls. The absolute differences between the pairs of
ages are similar in each sex until 7 years; later they
are generally greater in the girls than the boys.

The mean differences between RWT assessments of
the knee and Greulich-Pyle assessments of the hand-
wrist are given in Table XXXVII. The sample size at
each age varies from 15 to 135. The relative differences in the boys are near zero except from 5 through
8 years when the knee values are consistently the
higher by about 0.4 years. However, towards the end of
the scale (15 and 16 years), the mean ages for the knee
are about 0.4 years less than those for the hand-wrist.
The pattern of differences across age is similar in
the girls in whom the knee ages are the greater from
3 through 6 years by about 0.3 years but the difference
is in the opposite direction at 13 and 14 years when
the means of the values assigned to the hand-wrist are
about 0.4 years greater than those assigned to the knee.
These differences could be due to vagaries of sampling
either in the Brush Foundation Study or the Fels
Longitudinal Study, or both, but one would not expect
that this influence would be large because both studies
were "longitudinal" with, however, some missed visits.
The other possible factors are that the selection of
standards by Greulich and Pyle (1959) may have been
imperfect or that systematic errors were made when the
Greulich and Pyle standards were used to assess the
present group of radiographs. The mean absolute differences are larger in the boys than the girls at most
ages. These differences increase in each sex until
about 9 years after which only irregular and generally
small changes occur.

TABLE XXXVII

Mean Differences (Years) between RWT and
Greulich-Pyle Skeletal Ages (Knee and
Hand-Wrist, Respectively) for Children in
the Fels Longitudinal Study

Chronological	Relative		Absolute	
age	Boys	Girls	Boys	Girls
0.1	-0.37	-0.15	0.41	0.18
0.3	-0.13	-0.03	0.26	0.17
0.5	0.08	0.00	0.25	0.20
0.8	0.03	0.01	0.27	0.25
1.0	0.01	-0.08	0.36	0.25
1.5	0.01	0.01	0.29	0.30
2.0	0.10	0.10	0.32	0.32
2.5	0.14	0.18	0.38	0.36
3.0	0.14	0.29	0.39	0.50
3.5	0.19	0.32	0.47	0.56
4.0	0.10	0.37	0.48	0.71
4.5	0.38	0.29	0.62	0.57
5.0	0.45	0.34	0.77	0.63
5.5	0.39	0.40	0.74	0.57
6.0	0.41	0.27	0.75	0.60
6.5	0.30	0.16	0.69	0.62
7.0	0.41	0.25	0.71	0.67
7.5	0.06	0.35	0.64	0.78
8.0	0.44	0.23	0.76	0.68
8.5	0.09	-0.02	0.79	0.77
9.0	0.37	0.04	0.76	0.55
9.5	-0.12	-0.11	1.09	0.74
10.0	0.04	-0.01	0.77	0.79
11.0	-0.09	0.12	0.67	0.75
12.0	-0.24	0.02	0.76	0.60
13.0	0.09	-0.38	0.68	0.60
14.0	-0.11	-0.46	0.66	0.75
15.0	-0.38	----	0.65	----
16.0	-0.51	----	0.65	----

   A similar comparison was made between skeletal
ages obtained for the knee by the RWT method and by
the method of Tanner et al. (1962, 1972, 1975) for the
hand-wrist (Table XXXVIII).Those obtained by the method
of Tanner et al. are referred to as "Tanner-Whitehouse"
skeletal ages. The modified TWII system was used.
At all ages in each sex, except near the end of the
scale in the girls, the Tanner-Whitehouse skeletal
ages are greater than the RWT ages. These mean differences tend to increase with age in each sex until
about 7 years. After remaining approximately steady
for a few years, the mean differences tend to decrease
after 12 years in boys and 9.5 years in girls. It will
be recalled that, due to the statistical constraints
imposed during the construction of the present scale,
the mean RWT skeletal age is approximately equal to
the mean chronological age within each chronological
age group. Consequently, the present findings show
that the Tanner-Whitehouse levels are set too low for
this group of children. These findings are consistent
with earlier reports that, when the Greulich-Pyle and
Tanner-Whitehouse methods are each applied to the same
group of hand-wrist radiographs, the Greulich-Pyle
skeletal ages are systematically lower than the Tanner-
Whitehouse ones (Fry, 1966 and personal communication;
Asiel, 1966; Andersen, 1968; Roche et al., 1971; Blanco
et al., 1974). The absolute differences between pairs
of measurements obtained by these two methods are
similar in each sex until about 8 years; at later ages
they are greater in the boys than the girls until
14 years. The general trend in each sex is for these
differences to increase to 9 years after which they
decrease gradually and irregularly.

   Using these same data, correlation coefficients
were calculated and regression lines were fitted across
ages (Table XXXIX). When RWT skeletal ages are
regressed on Pyle-Hoerr ages, the intercept is close
to zero in each sex. The slope is close to unity in
the boys but somewhat lower in the girls. When the
RWT ages for the knee are regressed against Greulich-
Pyle skeletal ages for the hand-wrist,these intercepts

TABLE   XXXVIII

Mean Differences (Years) between RWT and
Tanner-Whitehouse Skeletal Ages (Knee
and Hand-Wrist, Respectively) for
Children in the Fels Longitudinal Study

Chronological age	Relative		Absolute	
	Boys	Girls	Boys	Girls
0.1	----	----	----	----
0.3	----	----	----	----
0.5	----	-0.43	----	0.43
0.8	-0.40	-0.43	0.52	0.44
1.0	-0.24	-0.32	0.36	0.38
1.5	-0.08	-0.30	0.34	0.40
2.0	-0.16	-0.21	0.39	0.49
2.5	-0.25	-0.34	0.52	0.51
3.0	-0.31	-0.34	0.56	0.68
3.5	-0.38	-0.47	0.64	0.75
4.0	-0.61	-0.50	0.83	0.81
4.5	-0.52	-0.73	0.84	0.88
5.0	-0.56	-0.74	0.90	1.01
5.5	-0.68	-0.88	1.01	0.96
6.0	-0.76	-1.04	1.06	1.17
6.5	-1.04	-1.20	1.27	1.28
7.0	-1.06	-1.27	1.21	1.34
7.5	-1.46	-0.99	1.48	1.23
8.0	-1.09	-1.12	1.23	1.18
8.5	-1.45	-1.28	1.51	1.38
9.0	-1.26	-1.03	1.37	1.04
9.5	-1.56	-1.03	1.70	1.17
10.0	-1.12	-0.93	1.20	1.08
11.0	-1.25	-0.72	1.33	0.84
12.0	-1.40	-0.80	1.46	0.94
13.0	-0.94	-0.75	1.01	0.82
14.0	-1.08	-0.45	1.11	0.79
15.0	-0.58	0.11	0.69	0.77
16.0	-0.83	0.19	0.95	0.67
17.0	-0.54	0.23	0.67	0.56

also are close to zero and the slopes are almost unity
in each sex. When Tanner-Whitehouse skeletal ages for
the hand-wrist are regressed against RWT skeletal ages
for the knee, the slope is close to one in each sex but
the intercept is about 0.7 years in the boys and 1.0
years in the girls indicating that the Tanner-Whitehouse
skeletal ages are systematically greater than the RWT
ages by considerable amounts; this difference is
greater in the girls. These data show that systematic
differences are present between Tanner-Whitehouse and
RWT skeletal ages when obtained for the same group of
radiographs. As noted earlier, several have reported
corresponding differences between Greulich-Pyle and
Tanner-Whitehouse skeletal ages. There is little doubt
that these differences are not due to variations in
the methods of weighting between the two systems.
Instead, they reflect true differences between the
upper socioeconomic class Cleveland children used as
a standardizing group by Greulich and Pyle and the
groups of Scottish children used for the same purpose

TABLE XXXIX

Values for regression lines and correlation
coefficients between various measures of skeletal age

	Boys			
	N	a	b	r
RWT v. PH	2057	0.07	0.99	+0.99
RWT v. GP	2701	0.01	0.98	+0.98
RWT v. TW	1454	0.69	1.03	+0.97
	Girls			
	N	a	b	r
RWT v. PH	1448	0.13	0.91	+0.98
RWT v. GP	2280	-0.04	0.98	+0.98
RWT v. TW	1376	1.01	0.97	+0.98

PH=Pyle and Hoerr; GP=Greulich and Pyle; TW=Tanner et al.

by Tanner and his colleagues (Roche et al., 1971).
Presumably a similar factor is responsible for the
systematic differences between the RWT and Tanner-
Whitehouse skeletal ages assigned to pairs of radiographs of the hand-wrist and knee taken of children at
single examinations.

When calculated across ages, the correlation
coefficients between the RWT and the other skeletal
ages were either +0.97 or +0.98 indicating an almost
exact relationship between these ages within each pair.
These coefficients are spurious, however, because of
the long chronological age range and the fact that,
with each system of assessment, skeletal age has an
approximately rectilinear relationship to chronological age. When one of these effects is removed by
calculating correlations within chronological age
groups, the coefficients are reduced markedly
(Tables XL and XLI) but, with the exception of
one age in the boys, all the coefficients remain positive and almost all are highly significant. Those
between RWT skeletal ages and Pyle and Hoerr skeletal
ages are about +0.6. Those between RWT and Greulich-
Pyle skeletal ages are lower, being generally in the
range +0.4 to +0.5. The fact that these values are
lower presumably reflects the fact that different
joints are being assessed; it is known that the
maturity levels of the hand-wrist and knee can vary
considerably within individuals (Todd, 1937; Garn
et al., 1961a, 1966a; Roche and French, 1970). The
correlations between RWT and Tanner-Whitehouse skeletal
ages tend to be at about the same levels as those with
Greulich-Pyle skeletal ages. The comparisons do not
show age-associated trends in the values of the
coefficients.

In the corresponding data for the girls also, the
correlation coefficients are generally highly
significant. In fact, they tend to be higher than
those for the boys. In each of the three comparisons,
there is no evidence of an age-associated trend in the
values of the coefficients. Those between the RWT and

TABLE   XL

Correlation coefficients between RWT
and other skeletal ages in boys

Chronological age	Pyle and Hoerr		Greulich and Pyle		Tanner-Whitehouse	
	N	r	N	r	N	r
0.1	40	.42**	6	---	---	---
0.3	60	.45**	35	.32	---	---
0.5	98	.46**	84	.42**	1	---
0.8	67	.06	68	.28*	7	-.02
1.0	98	.30*	122	.20*	29	.16
1.5	97	.55**	96	.53**	44	.34*
2.0	124	.61**	134	.44**	52	.47**
2.5	91	.62**	96	.39**	54	.43**
3.0	106	.70**	134	.42**	60	.50**
3.5	88	.57**	91	.45**	63	.51**
4.0	114	.67**	132	.44**	62	.54**
4.5	92	.55**	95	.46**	72	.50**
5.0	121	.60**	127	.52**	72	.48**
5.5	79	.57**	82	.55**	65	.42**
6.0	115	.62**	135	.47**	70	.43**
6.5	7	.90**	98	.48**	58	.49**
7.0	117	.65**	134	.53**	75	.51**
7.5	1	---	91	.34**	60	.56**
8.0	106	.61**	127	.44**	73	.53**
8.5	2	---	93	.38**	64	.50**
9.0	85	.63**	123	.55**	69	.53**
9.5	2	---	46	.47**	39	.54**
10.0	84	.60**	114	.40**	68	.49**
11.0	73	.56**	101	.58**	56	.58**
12.0	67	.63**	96	.52**	53	.66**
13.0	63	.71**	98	.62**	51	.80**
14.0	49	.50**	92	.64**	44	.70**
15.0	36	.48**	42	.64**	34	.72**
16.0	13	.38	16	.39	33	.71**
17.0	3	---	3	---	37	.51**
18.0	---	---	---	---	20	.54*

* = P < .05   ** = P < .01.

TABLE XLI

Correlation coefficients between RWT
and other skeletal ages in girls

Chronological age	Pyle and Hoerr		Greulich and Pyle		Tanner-Whitehouse	
	N	r	N	r	N	r
0.1	4	---	19	.41	---	---
0.3	5	---	66	.33**	1	---
0.5	13	.62*	99	.40**	4	---
0.8	8	.90**	91	.38**	12	.73**
1.0	24	.49*	109	.35**	31	.53**
1.5	84	.69**	102	.24*	54	.44**
2.0	97	.56**	109	.49**	52	.43**
2.5	85	.80**	93	.55**	58	.60**
3.0	112	.65**	124	.58**	67	.62**
3.5	87	.84**	92	.60**	63	.57**
4.0	92	.76**	111	.58**	67	.62**
4.5	75	.83**	80	.68**	64	.67**
5.0	105	.73**	117	.64**	68	.58**
5.5	64	.83**	67	.71**	55	.75**
6.0	101	.63**	119	.66**	71	.62**
6.5	2	---	79	.60**	54	.48**
7.0	94	.65**	122	.52**	70	.63**
7.5	1	---	79	.46**	59	.36**
8.0	80	.71**	104	.63**	64	.57**
8.5	12	.71**	80	.61**	58	.56**
9.0	76	.69**	104	.72**	66	.64**
9.5	6	---	75	.40**	64	.51**
10.0	76	.59**	109	.52**	65	.58**
11.0	64	.49**	87	.64**	54	.67**
12.0	65	.54**	81	.58**	53	.58**
13.0	41	.69**	52	.44**	41	.62**
14.0	40	.65**	15	.26	43	.66**
15.0	19	.66**	4	---	33	.68**
16.0	6	---	---	---	35	.53
17.0	2	---	---	---	14	.18
18.0	---	---	---	---	9	---

*= P < .05   ** = P < .01.

Pyle-Hoerr skeletal ages, each of the knee, are about
+0.7; those between RWT and either Greulich-Pyle or
Tanner-Whitehouse skeletal ages are about +0.6. As
noted earlier for boys, it is reasonable to assume
that the coefficients between RWT and Pyle-Hoerr
ratings tend to be the higher because the same area is
being assessed with each method.

ABNORMAL CHILDREN

An analysis was made of the applicability of the
RWT method to children with pathological conditions
that could have affected the rates and/or patterns of
maturation at the knee joint. For this purpose,
assessments were made of 72 radiographs of 18 children
ranging in age from 1 month to 17.7 years. At the
time of radiography, these children were suffering
from poliomyelitis, hypophosphatasia, hypothyroidism,
Gaucher's disease, Hurler's syndrome, osteomyelitis
of the knee, chondromatosis, osteochondritis of the
patella or fibula, osteochondritis dissecans, or
osteogenesis imperfecta.

All the radiographs could be assessed. The
standard errors of the estimate are generally near the
median values for normal children at the same chronological ages with a few exceptions in which the standard errors deviate from the median values in either
direction but are within the range from the tenth to
the ninetieth percentile. These findings show the
RWT method is as effective in the assessment of these
abnormal children as it is in normal children. This
finding is, of course, very important in relation to
the clinical application of the new method.

CHAPTER VIII

SUMMARY AND CONCLUSIONS

It is well known that children of the same chronological age and sex differ in maturity levels. These differences occur in all body systems but the skeletal system is assessed more frequently than others mainly because these assessments can be made during a wide age range and because skeletal maturity levels are known to have general significance for the growth and development of the body. Despite this, if the maturity level of a particular body system, other than the skeleton, is required, this should be assessed directly and not inferred from skeletal age. However, few other systems can be assessed with a useful level of accuracy.

Skeletal age assessments are needed for the clinical management of children with chromosomal or endocrine abnormalities and those who are unusual in stature, to predict adult statures and to select ages for surgically induced epiphyseal fusion. In the past, the hand-wrist area has been assessed more often than others. However, the knee is a preferable area because it is more closely related to stature; this is important because, at least in clinical circumstances, assessments of skeletal maturity are needed commonly in children with deviant statures. In addition, the knee has advantages over the hand-wrist in the length of the interval during which it can be assessed and the absence of long age ranges during which maturational changes cannot be observed. A summary of the previous literature relating to scales of skeletal maturity and the changes that occur during the maturation of the knee are presented.

251

Usually skeletal maturity is assessed by the atlas method. In this system, the radiograph to be assessed is compared with a series of standards derived from normal children. When this procedure is applied, maturity indicators are observed but not recorded and data from these indicators are combined subjectively by the assessor to obtain a skeletal age expressed in years and months.

The Pyle and Hoerr atlas for the knee contains a series of standard plates that show the central tendencies for maturity level in a group of privileged Cleveland children. Problems with the atlas method concern the need for both anteroposterior and lateral radiographs (and thus more irradiation), the provision of a single set of standards (thereby failing to provide a range of shapes at the same maturity level), and the lack of a standardized methodology by which assessments should be made and bone-specific skeletal ages combined (leading to increased inter-observer differences). Finally, the Pyle and Hoerr atlas does not provide data relating to the normal range of skeletal ages within chronological age groups and, as noted earlier, the atlas method cannot provide the error of the estimate for an individual radiograph.

The Pyle and Hoerr atlas provides a single set of standards for both sexes. Differences in the sequence of maturity indicators (limited, however, to onset of ossification and epiphyseo-diaphyseal fusion) between the sexes have been reported for some skeletal areas. An analysis of the very large body of data recorded during the present investigation showed that sex-associated differences in sequence in the knee were very slight. This shows Pyle and Hoerr were justified in combining the sex-specific standards in their 1955 atlas to a unisex series in the 1969 atlas.

The RWT method was developed using data from about 8,000 serial radiographs of 552 "normal" children who were generally of middle socioeconomic level. The radiographs had been taken between 1932 and 1972 but there were no real secular trends in the maturity levels

of these radiographs. This was demonstrated by corre-
lating RWT skeletal ages with year of birth and by
comparing skeletal ages, within parent-offspring pairs,
for radiographs taken at the same chronological age.

Lists of possible indicators were compiled from
the literature and their descriptions were made simple
and clear. Effective objective methods were developed
for grading these indicators. Those based on the curvature of margins were graded by fitting constructed
curves; some others were based on measurements or the
fitting of straight lines. This emphasis on indicators
was necessary because one aim was to develop a method
in which the replicability of skeletal age assessments
was independent of variant sequences of maturation
among and within bones.

Indicators were accepted as useful only if they
discriminated, became universal, were reliable and were
valid and could be observed in all, or almost all, the
radiographs, within particular age ranges. As expected,
the useful age ranges differed among indicators.
Prevalence data for each grade of the useful indicators
were graphed on probability paper. These allowed
approximate estimates of the ages at which the grades
were reached in 50 percent of the group (thresholds) and
judgments of the rates of change in prevalence with age.
The more rapid this change the more informative the
indicator. Also, these graphs showed the regularity of
changes in prevalence across age and the age ranges
during which each indicator grade would be useful.

To combine data from the useful indicators, continuous variables (ratios) were changed to categories.
The ordered categories for these and other indicators
were combined to a single continuous index, using a
latent trait analysis for the multiple graded case.
The scaling was set so that the mean and variance of
skeletal age were equal to the mean and the variance
of chronological age in the sample. This statistical
method separates the within age variance to the real
variation in actual maturity levels and the variation
due to error. The latter element is due partly to

inaccurate recording but reflects also the limited
ability of available indicators to provide all of the
information about the level of skeletal maturity.

The RWT method for the assessment of the knee is
based on standardized procedures, and is applicable to
a single anteroposterior radiograph over a wide range
of maturity levels. It provides a range of shapes for
indicators at the same maturity level and utilizes all
the useful information coded from each radiograph.
When the new RWT method is used, there is an increase
in validity, an increase in the proportion of individuals who can be assessed at each end of the chronological age range and it provides the error of the
estimate for each radiograph, which no other current
method can do.

The RWT method of assessment is applied by grading
particular indicators, depending on age and sex. These
data are transferred to a small computer in which a
skeletal age estimation program (Appendix II) is stored.
The computer output provides the skeletal age in years,
together with the standard error of this estimate.
If some indicators appropriate for age and sex are not
graded, the skeletal age assigned will be less accurate
as will be clear from the large standard error of the
estimate. Sets of test radiographs, together with the
grades assigned to them, are available to assist the
training of new assessors. The RWT method can be
expanded easily to encompass additional indicators
and/or sites without costly renorming. This is accomplished by scoring the new indicators, using the same
latent trait model and standardizing them to chronological age. The usefulness of such an enterprise will
be shown by the reduction in the standard errors.

BIBLIOGRAPHY

Abbott, O. D., R. O. Townsend, R. B. French and C. F. Ahmann 1950 Carpal and epiphysial development. Another index of nutritional status of rural school children. Am. J. Dis. Child., 79: 69-81.

Acheson, R. M. 1954 A method of assessing skeletal maturity from radiographs. A report from the Oxford Child Health Survey. J. Anat. (Lond.), 88: 498-508.

———————————— 1966 Maturation of the skeleton. In: Human Development. F. Falkner, ed. W. B. Saunders Co., Philadelphia, pp. 465-502.

Acheson, R. M., and C. W. Dupertuis 1957 The relationship between physique and rate of skeletal maturation in boys. Hum. Biol., 29: 167-193.

Acheson, R. M., G. Fowler, E. I. Fry, M. Janes, K. Koski, P. Urbano and J. J. Van der Werff Ten Bosch 1963 Studies in the reliability of assessing skeletal maturity from X-rays. Greulich-Pyle Atlas, Part I. Hum. Biol., 35: 317-349.

Adair, F. L., and R. E. Scammon 1921 Ossification centers of the wrist, knee and ankle at birth, with particular reference to the physical development and maturity of the new born. Am. J. Obstr. & Gyn., 2: 35-60.

Aitchison, J., and S. D. Silvey 1957 The generalization of probit analysis to the case of multiple responses. Biometrika, 44: 131-140.

255

Andersen, E.   1968   Skeletal Maturation of Danish
    School Children in Relation to Height, Sexual
    Development, and Social Conditions.   Acta paediat.
    Scandinav., Suppl. 185, pp. 133.

———————————— 1971 Comparison of Tanner-Whitehouse
    and Greulich-Pyle methods in a large scale Danish
    survey. Am. J. Phys. Anthrop., 35: 373-376.

Anderson, M.   1967   Growth, overgrowth, and maturity:
    observations based upon examination of serial
    roentgenograms of children with hemihypertrophy.
    Am. J. Phys. Anthrop., 27: 246.

———————————— 1971   Use of the Greulich-Pyle "Atlas
    of Skeletal Development of the Hand and Wrist" in
    a clinical context. Am. J. Phys. Anthrop., 35:
    347-351.

Anderson, M., S.-C. Hwang and W. T. Green 1965   Growth
    of the normal trunk in boys and girls during the
    second decade of life, related to age, maturity,
    and ossification of the iliac epiphyses. J. Bone
    & Jt. Surg., 47A: 1554-1564.

Asiel, M.   1966   Considérations sur l'utilisation des
    méthodes de Greulich et Pyle et de Tanner pour
    l'évaluation de la maturation osseuse d'un
    échantillon de garçons agés de cinq à neuf ans.
    In: Compte Rendu de la Réunion des Equipes
    Chargées des Etudes sur la Croissance et le
    Développment de l'Enfant Normal, Stockholm.
    Centre International de l'Enfance, Paris, 1: 53-59.

Baer, M. J., and J. Durkatz 1957 Bilateral asymmetry
    in skeletal maturation of hand and wrist: roentgeno-
    graphic analysis. Am. J. Phys. Anthrop., 15:
    181-196.

Baldwin, B. T., L. M. Busby and H. V. Garside 1928
    Anatomic Growth of Children. A Study of Some
    Bones of the Hand, Wrist and Lower Forearm by
    Means of Roentgenograms. Univ. Iowa Stud. Child
    Welfare, 4: No. 1, pp. 88.

Bardeen, C. R.   1921   The relation of ossification to
    physiological development. J. Radiol., 2: 1-8.

Bayer, L. M., and R. R. Newell   1940   The assessment of
    skeletal development of the hand and knee between
    the ages of 8 and 14 years. Endocrinology, 26:
    779-782.

Bayley, N.   1943   Skeletal maturing in adolescence as
    a basis for determining percentage of completed
    growth. Child Develop., 14: 1-46.

——————————————   1962   The accurate prediction of growth
    and adult height. Mod. Probl. Paediat., 7: 234-255.

Bayley, N., and S. R. Pinneau   1952   Tables for predict-
    ing adult height from skeletal age: revised for
    use with Greulich-Pyle hand standards. J. Pediat.,
    40: 423-441.

Berkson, J.   1951   Why I prefer logits to probits.
    Biometrics, 7: 327-339.

——————————————   1955   Maximum likelihood and minimum
    chi-square estimates of the logistic function. J.
    Am. Statis. Assn., 50: 130-162.

Birnbaum, A.   1968   Some latent trait models and their
    use in inferring an examinee's ability.   In:
    Statistical Theories of Mental Test Scores.
    F. M. Lord and M. R. Novick, eds. Addison-Wesley,
    Reading, Mass., Chapters 17-20.

Blanco, R. A., R. M. Acheson, C. Canosa and J. B.
    Solomon   1974   Height, weight and lines of
    arrested growth in young Guatemalan children.
    Am. J. Phys. Anthrop., 40: 39-48.

Bock, R. D.   1972   Estimating item parameters and
    latent ability when responses are scored in two or
    more nominal categories. Psychometrika, 37: 29-51.

Bock, R. D., and R. Wood 1971 Test theory. Ann. Rev. Psych., 22: 193-224.

Borovanský, L., and O. Hněvkovský 1929 The growth of the body and the process of ossification in Prague boys from 4 years to 19 years. Anthropologie (Prague), 7: 169-208.

Brožek, J. 1956 Body Measurements and Human Nutrition. Wayne University Press, Detroit, pp. 167.

Brunk, U., and G. Sköld 1962 Length of foetus and ossification of the toe and finger phalanges. Acta Histochem. (Jena), 14: 59-66.

Caffey, J., H. M. Samuel, C. Royer and P. Morales 1958 Ossification of the distal femoral epiphysis. J. Bone & Jt. Surg., 40A: 647-654.

Carlos, J. P., and A. M. Gittelsohn 1965 Longitudinal studies of the natural history of caries. I. Eruption patterns of the permanent teeth. J. Dent. Res., 44: 509-516.

Cheek, D. B., R. B. Schultz, A. Parra and R. C. Reba 1970 Overgrowth of lean and adipose tissues in adolescent obesity. Pediat. Res., 4: 268-279.

Christ, H. H. 1961 A discussion of causes of error in the determination of chronological age in children by means of x-ray studies of carpal-bone development. S. Afr. Med. J., 35: 854-857.

Christ, N. 1929 Über die endochondrale Ossifications Zone der distalen Femurepiphyse. Arch. f. Orthop. u. Unfall. Chir., 27: 610-630.

Clarke, H. H., and E. W. Degutis 1962 Comparison of skeletal age and various physical and motor factors with the pubescent development of 10, 13, and 16 year old boys. Res. Quart., 33: 356-368.

Clarke, H. H., and N. R. Hayman   1962   Reduction of
    bone assessments necessary for the skeletal age
    determination of boys.   Res. Quart., 33: 202-207.

Clements, E. M. B., E. Davies-Thomas and K. G. Pickett
    1953   Time of eruption of permanent teeth in
    Bristol children in 1947-48.   Brit. Med. J., i:
    1421-1424.

Cohn, I.   1922   Observations on the normally developing
    knee.   Arch. Surg., 5: 395-412.

Crampton, C. W.   1908   Physiological age--a fundamental
    principle.   Am. Phys. Educ. Rev., 13.   Reprinted
    in Child Develop., 1944, 15: 3-51.

Crandall, V. C.   1972   The Fels Study: Some contribu-
    tions to personality development and achievement
    in childhood and adulthood.   Seminars Psychiat.,
    4: 383-397.

Dedick, A. P., and J. Caffey   1953   Roentgen findings
    in the skull and chest in 1,030 newborn infants.
    Radiology, 61: 13-20.

Demirjian, A., and H. Goldstein   1972   A new system of
    dental age assessment.   In: Compte-Rendu de la
    XIe Réunion des Equipes Chargées des Etudes sur
    la Croissance et le Développement de L'Enfant
    Normal, Londres.   Centre International de
    L'Enfance, Paris, p. 137.

Demirjian, A., H. Goldstein and J. M. Tanner   1973
    A new system of dental age assessment.   Hum. Biol.,
    45: 211-227.

Demisch, A., and P. Wartmann   1956   Calcification of
    mandibular third molar and its relation to
    skeletal and chronological age in children.
    Child Develop., 27: 459-473.

Gardner, E., and D. J. Gray 1953 Prenatal development of the human shoulder and acromioclavicular joints. Am. J. Anat., 92: 219-276.

Gardner, E., D. J. Gray and R. O'Rahilly 1959 The prenatal development of the skeleton and joints of the human foot. J. Bone & Jt. Surg., 41A: 847-876.

Garn, S. M., and Y. French 1967 Magnitude of secular trend in the Fels population: stature; weight. Privately printed.

Garn, S. M., and C. G. Rohmann 1959 Communalities of the ossification centers of the hand and wrist. Am. J. Phys. Anthrop., 17: 319-323.

——————— 1960 Variability in the order of ossification of the bony centers of the hand and wrist. Am. J. Phys. Anthrop., 18: 219-230.

Garn, S. M., A. B. Lewis and D. W. Shoemaker 1956 The sequence of calcification of the mandibular molar and pre-molar teeth. J. Dent. Res., 35: 555-561.

Garn, S. M., C. G. Rohmann and M. Robinow 1961 Increments in hand-wrist ossification. Am. J. Phys. Anthrop., 19: 45-53.

Garn, S. M., C. G. Rohmann and B. Apfelbaum 1961a Complete epiphyseal union of the hand. Am. J. Phys. Anthrop., 19: 365-372.

Garn, S. M., C. G. Rohmann and D. K. Wallace 1961b Association between alternate sequences of hand-wrist ossification. Am. J. Phys. Anthrop., 19: 361-364.

Garn, S. M., F. N. Silverman and C. G. Rohmann 1964 A rational approach to the assessment of skeletal maturation. Ann. Radiol., 7: 297-307.

Garn, S. M., C. G. Rohmann and T. Blumenthal   1966
     Ossification sequence polymorphism and sexual
     dimorphism in skeletal development. Am. J. Phys.
     Anthrop., 24: 101-115.

Garn, S. M., C. G. Rohmann, T. Blumenthal and C. S.
     Kaplan   1966a   Developmental communalities of
     homologous and non-homologous body joints. Am. J.
     Phys. Anthrop., 25: 147-151.

Garn, S. M., C. G. Rohmann and F. N. Silverman   1967
     Radiographic standards for postnatal ossification
     and tooth calcification. Med. Radiogr. & Photogr.,
     43: 45-66.

Garn, S. M., C. G. Rohmann, T. Blumenthal and F. N.
     Silverman   1967a   Ossification communalities of
     the hand and other body parts: Their implication
     to skeletal assessment. Am. J. Phys. Anthrop.,
     27: 75-82.

Garn, S. M., A. K. Poznanski and J. M. Nagy   1971   The
     operational meaning of maturity criteria. Am. J.
     Phys. Anthrop., 35: 319-326.

Gleiser, I., and E. E. Hunt, Jr.   1955   The permanent
     mandibular first molar: its calcification, eruption
     and decay. Am. J. Phys. Anthrop., 13: 253-284.

Goldstein, H.   1975   Personal communication.

Gray, D. J., and E. J. Gardner   1950   Prenatal develop-
     ment of the human knee and superior tibiofibular
     joints. Am. J. Anat., 86: 235-287.

Gray, D. J., E. Gardner and R. O'Rahilly   1957   The
     prenatal development of the skeleton and joints
     of the human hand. Am. J. Anat., 101: 169-223.

Gray, S. W., and F. P. Lamons   1959   Skeletal develop-
     ment and tooth eruption in Atlanta children.
     Am. J. Orthod., 45: 272-277.

Greulich, W. W. 1954 The relationship of skeletal
    status to the physical growth and development of
    children. In: Dynamics of Growth Processes.
    E. J. Boell, ed. Princeton University Press,
    Princeton, pp. 212-223.

Greulich, W., and S. I. Pyle 1950 Radiographic Atlas
    of Skeletal Development of the Hand and Wrist.
    Stanford University Press, Stanford, Calif.,
    pp. 190.

_____ 1959 Radiographic Atlas of Skeletal
    Development of the Hand and Wrist, 2nd Ed. Stan-
    ford University Press, Stanford, Calif., pp. 256.

Hadley, L. A. 1956 The Spine. Anatomico-Radiographic
    Studies: Development and the Cervical Region.
    Charles C Thomas, Springfield, Ill., pp. 156.

Haines, R. W., and A. Mohiuddin 1959 A preliminary
    note on the process of epiphysial union. J. Fac.
    Med., Baghdad, 1: 141-147.

_____ 1962 Epiphysial growth and union in
    the pigeon. J. Fac. Med., Baghdad, 4: 4-21.

Ham, A. W. 1969 Histology. 6th Ed. Lippincott,
    Philadelphia, pp. 1037.

Hansman, C. F. 1962 Appearance and fusion of ossifi-
    cation centers in the human skeleton. Am. J.
    Roentgenol., 88: 476-482.

Hansman, C. F., and M. M. Maresh 1961 A longitudinal
    study of skeletal maturation. Am. J. Dis. Child.,
    101: 305-321.

Hartley, J. B. 1957 Radiological estimation of foetal
    maturity. Brit. J. Radiol., 30: 561-576.

Hayman, N. R. 1959 Reduction of the Number of Bone
    Assessments Necessary for Skeletal Age Determina-
    tion of Adolescent Boys. Microcard, Doctoral
    Dissertation, University of Oregon.

Healy, M. J. R., and H. Goldstein. The scaling of
    categorical response data. Unpublished.

Hellman, M. 1928 Ossification of epiphyseal cartilages
    in the hand. Am. J. Phys. Anthrop., 11: 223-257.

Heřt, J. 1972 Growth of the epiphyseal plate in cir-
    cumference. Acta Anat., 82: 420-436.

Hesser, C. 1926 Beitrag zur Kenntnis der Gelenkent-
    wicklung beim Menschen. Morph. Jahrb., 55: 489-567.

Hewitt, D., and R. M. Acheson 1961 Some aspects of
    skeletal development through adolescence.
    I. Variations in the rate and pattern of skeletal
    maturation at puberty. Am. J. Phys. Anthrop.,
    19: 321-331.

———————————— 1961a Some aspects of skeletal develop-
    ment through adolescence. II. The interrelation-
    ship between skeletal maturation and growth at
    puberty. Am. J. Phys. Anthrop., 19: 333-344.

Hewitt, D., C. K. Westropp and R. M. Acheson 1955
    Oxford Child Health Survey. Effect of childish
    ailments on skeletal development. Brit. J. Prev.
    & Soc. Med., 9: 179-186.

Hill, A. F. 1939 Fetal age assessment by centers of
    ossification. Am. J. Phys. Anthrop., 24: 251-272.

Hoerr, N. L., S. I. Pyle and C. C. Francis 1962
    Radiographic Atlas of Skeletal Development of the
    Foot and Ankle. A Standard of Reference. Charles
    C Thomas, Springfield, Ill., pp. 163.

Hogben, H., J. A. H. Waterhouse and L. Hogben 1948
    Studies on puberty, Part I. Brit. J. Soc. Med.,
    2:29-42.

Howard, C. C.   1928   The physiologic progress of the
     bone centers of the hands of normal children
     between the ages of five and sixteen inclusive;
     also a comparative study of both retarded and
     accelerated hand growth in children whose general
     growth is similarly affected.   Int. J. Orthod.,
     14: 948-997.

Hughes, P. C. R., and J. M. Tanner   1970   The assess-
     ment of skeletal maturity in the growing rat. J.
     Anat., 106: 371-402.

Hunt, E. E., Jr., G. Cocke and J. R. Gallagher   1958
     Somatotype and sexual maturation in boys: A method
     of developmental analysis.   Hum. Biol., 30: 73-91.

Hurme, V. O.   1949   Ranges of normalcy in the eruption
     of the permanent teeth.   J. Dent. Child., 16:
     11-15.

Ingalls, N. W.   1927   Studies on the femur; the femur
     at birth.   Am. J. Phys. Anthrop., 11: 107-121.

Jackson, R. L.   1966   Effect of malnutrition on growth
     of the pre-school child.   In: Pre-school Child
     Malnutrition; Primary Deterrent to Human Progress.
     Pub. No. 1282, Natl. Acad. Sci., Nat. Res. Council,
     Washington, D.C., pp. 9-21.

Jelliffe, D. B.   1966   The Assessment of the Nutritional
     Status of the Community.   W.H.O. Monograph No. 53,
     Geneva, pp. 271.

Johnson, L. C.   1966   The kinetics of skeletal remodel-
     ing; structural organization of the skeleton.
     Birth Defects, Original Article Ser., 11: 66-142.

Johnston, F. E.   1963   Skeletal age and its prediction
     in Philadelphia children.   Hum. Biol., 35: 192-201.

Johnston, F. E., and S. B. Jahina   1965   The contribution
     of the carpal bones to the assessment of skeletal
     age.   Am. J. Phys. Anthrop., 23: 349-354.

McKern,
    Cl
    St
    Re
    D:
    De
    pr

Macy, 1
    Cl
    Tl

Macy, 1
    po
    Ur

Mainlar
    me
    Il
    ge

Malcolm
    Gu
    Di
    Bi

Malina,
    Se
    Ur
    Se
    St

Maresh,
    lo
    fa
    du
    28

    of
    Ph

Jones, H. E. 1949 Motor Performance and Growth.
    A Developmental Study of Static Dynamometric
    Strength. University of California Press,
    Berkeley, pp. 182.

Joss, E. E., E. H. Sobel and K. A. Zuppinger 1963
    Skeletal maturation in rats with special reference
    to order and time of epiphysial closure. Endo-
    crinology, 72: 117-122.

Kelly, H. J., and I. G. Macy 1958 Roentgenographic
    appraisals of skeletal growth and development.
    Reliability and influencing factors. Am. J.
    Roentgenol., 80: 482-494.

Kelly, H. J., and L. Reynolds 1947 Appearance and
    growth of ossification centers and increases in
    the body dimensions of White and Negro infants.
    Am. J. Roentgenol., 57: 477-516.

Kessler, A., and R. B. Scott 1950 Growth and develop-
    ment of negro infants. II. Relation of birth
    weight, body length and epiphysial maturation to
    economic status. Am. J. Dis. Child., 80: 370-378.

Kihlberg, J., and K. Koski 1954 On the properties of
    the tooth eruption curve. Finska Tandläksällak.
    Forh., 50: 6-10.

Köhler, A., and E. A. Zimmer 1968 Borderlands of the
    Normal and Early Pathologic in Skeletal Roent-
    genology. 11th Rev. Ed., Grune and Stratton,
    New York, pp. 646.

Kolakowski, D., and R. D. Bock 1973 LOGOG: Maximum
    Likelihood Item Analysis and Test Scoring-Logistic
    Model for Multiple Item Responses. User's Guide.
    National Educational Resources, Inc., Ann Arbor,
    Mich., pp. 38.

———————————— 1972 A forty-five year investigation for secular changes in physical maturation. Am. J. Phys. Anthrop., 36: 103-110.

Mazess, R. B., and J. R. Cameron 1971 Skeletal growth in school children: Maturation and bone mass. Am. J. Phys. Anthrop., 35: 399-407.

Menees, T. O., and L. E. Holly 1932 Ossification in the extremities of the new-born. Am. J. Roentgenol., 28: 389-390.

Meredith, H. V. 1946 Order and age of eruption for the deciduous dentition. J. Dent. Res., 25: 43-66.

Meyer, D. B., and R. O'Rahilly 1958 Multiple techniques in the study of the onset of prenatal ossification. Anat. Rec., 132: 181-193.

Moed, G., B. W. Wight and H. N. Vandegrift 1962 Studies of physical disability: reliability of measurement of skeletal age from hand films. Child Develop., 33: 37-41.

Moss, M. L., and C. R. Noback 1958 A longitudinal study of digital epiphyseal fusion in adolescence. Anat. Rec., 131: 19-32.

Mossberg, H.-O. 1949 The X-ray appearance of the knee joint in obese overgrown children. Acta paediat. Scandinav., 38: 509-516.

Murray, J. R., R. D. Bock and A. F. Roche 1971 The measurement of skeletal maturity. Am. J. Phys. Anthrop., 35: 327-330.

Nicholson, A. B., and C. Hanley 1953 Indices of physiological maturity: derivation and interrelationships. Child Develop., 24: 3-38.